Mind Force Hypnosis:

Compiled By A. Thomas Perhacs

Published by Velocity Group Publishing

PO Box 9516 Hamilton, NJ 08650   www.advancedmindpower.com   www.mindforcesecrets.com

Introduction

DISCLAIMER

Neither A. Thomas Perhacs nor Velocity Group Publishing assumes any responsibility for the use or misuse of the concepts, methods and strategies contained in this book. The reader is warned that the use of some or all of the techniques in this book may result in legal consequences, civil and/or criminal.

USE OF THIS BOOK IS DONE AT YOUR OWN RISK.

(Updated Version, August 2008)

The books contained in this manuscript are used a bonus books to enhance your learning of Hypnosis. They should fill in the gaps to your learning and allow you to increase your knowledge profoundly.

A Thomas Perhacs

Hamilton, New Jersey

August, 2008

Table Of Contents

Hetero Hypnosis

Published by Velocity Group Publishing

PO Box 9516 Hamilton, NJ 08650   www.advancedmindpower.com   www.mindforcesecrets.com
© Copyright 2008   All Rights Reserved

Preliminary Remarks

Anyone can learn to hypnotize. At first glance hypnotizing may seem extremely simple. Any individual capable of memorizing and reciting a pattern of words can "learn" to hypnotize *some* individuals to *some* degree. Trance induction depends very little on the physical presence of a hypnotist. It is quite possible to induce hypnosis by playing a recording, containing the proper suggestions, to a person who has never met or seen the hypnotist. This is not to say that *all* individuals can be hypnotized in this manner or that a deep trance will be induced.

To master the skill of hypnosis, or any skill, there are three basic requirements. 1. Receiving competent instruction. 2. Acquiring practical experience, preferably under supervision. 3. Acquiring knowledge in related fields. Ideally hypnosis can best be learned in a university or school that provides a lecture-laboratory course, with combined practice sessions. Unfortunately there are few universities or schools offering such courses and those that do exist are geographically inaccessible to many students.

Keeping the above in mind, I have tried to write the following modules in such a way they will serve the needs of the beginner as well as the more advanced students of hypnotism.

Most students of hypnotism have learned to hypnotize by trial and error and the rote memorizing of stereotyped procedures with little opportunity to gain an understanding of what they are doing. I have tried to construct this course in such a way that it will give the student a working understanding of hypnosis and hypnotic phenomena. One of the fundamental premises of this work is that the only way to learn how to hypnotize effectively is through actual practice. I have therefore tried to present many of the techniques of hypnotism in the form of demonstrative experiments to be carried out by the student. These experiments have been carefully chosen to illustrate various fundamental concepts, bring out important facts, and offer the student actual practice. To make the text as much as possible a substitute for actual classroom instruction the basic demonstrations have been described in great detail. The student is told exactly, word for word, what to say, when to say it,and how to say it.

The objective of the following modules is to give the student the optimum training possible outside of a classroom. The reader should proceed in order from module to module and from exercise (experiment) to exercise. The student is strongly advised to keep going back over earlier material as he progresses and re-examine it in the light of his newly acquired experience. It is very important to first learn the waking suggestion techniques and experiments as presented in modules five through eight.

The modern sensorimotor method of inducing hypnosis is based entirely upon waking suggestions.

No matter how comprehensive a book may be there are certain things that can only be gained from long practice and experience. You can be become acquainted with the basic techniques of inducing hypnosis in a relative short period of time and with a minimum of effort, but it takes many years and hundreds of subjects to assimilate and master all the techniques of hypnosis. One of the most important factors in inducing hypnosis is self-confidence. This rarely comes from reading a "how-to-do-it" book. It is a by-product of repeated success, and learning through sheer experience.

Module 1 -- BEHAVIOR

In this module we will present some definitions of terms and concepts so there will be no misunderstanding as what is meant when these terms and concepts are encounter throughout the following modules.

BEHAVIOR

For our purposes we will define behavior as follows: Any observable activity of muscles or glands, such as movements of parts of the body, appearance of tears, perspiration, saliva and so forth. A smile is a behavior; so is talking, a grimace, trembling, blushing (produced by muscular changes in blood vessels), postural changes, eye movement as one follows words on a printed page.

MIND AND MENTAL ACTIVITY

By mind and mental activity we mean a function of the brain and nervous system in the same sense that digestion is a function of the stomach and gastrointestinal track; and circulation is a function of the heart and vascular system. All of the infinitely complex manifestations of cerebral activity can be ultimately reduced to two phenomena -- muscular movements and glandular discharges. Whether it is Einstein solving mathematical equations on a piece of paper, a child hugging a new toy or crying over the loss of a toy, a musician composing the next hit song or the president delivering his State of the Union speech -- all ultimately are manifestations of muscular movement and glandular changes. The end result of all mental activity is muscular movement and or glandular changes. At first thought this may seem wrong. In order to help you reconcile yourself to this idea, I would remind you that most people would agree that all cerebral activity is manifested by "words" and "actions." Under action, falls all external mechanical activity of which man is capable. Actions are only possible by using muscles. We use words to express ideas and communicate with one another. Words are sounds produced in the larynx and in the mouth cavity by muscular movement, unless they are written, in which case the muscles of the fingers are used. Therefore, *all external manifestations of the functioning of the brain can be reduced to muscular movement and a change in the secretions of the glands.* This includes such observable phenomena described as animation, joy, passion, sorrow, etc., which are the results of greater or lesser contractions of definite sets of muscles and glandular secretions such as tears. If it were not for our muscles, we could accomplish absolutely nothing. The muscles of our body are controlled by our brain and nervous system.

A TWO WAY STREET

Brain processes affect what happens in other organs of our body. Also, changes in other organs of the body in turn affect what happens in the brain. For example, anger or fear interrupts digestion, accelerates the beating of the heart, and increases the discharge of some glandular substances. The brain is not isolated from the rest of the body, how it functions depends on chemical substances delivered to it by the blood stream. The brain and the rest of the body constitute one system. Disorders in behavior may occur as a result of chemical changes in the body. They can also result from a person's perceptions and thoughts. We will have more to say about this later.

For our purposes we will divide human behavior into four categories:

1. **Voluntary Behavior**
2. **Nonvoluntary Behavior**
3. **Involuntary Behavior**
4. **Hypnotic Behavior**

By **voluntary behavior** we mean some action carried out by an individual, after he or she has made a conscious decision to perform the act. For example, If there should be a cup of coffee to the left of me on a table, but I feel I would rather have the coffee at my right, pick up the cup and move it to the right side of the table; I have performed a voluntary act. In order for an act to be voluntary, the individual performing the act must always know what is going to occur before the action takes place. In the above example, first there is the thought, "I would like to have the cup of coffee at my right." Next I decide to move the cup of coffee. Then I carry out the physical act of moving the coffee.

By **nonvoluntary behavior** we mean an action carried out by an individual that he or she did not consciously initiate, but once the individual becomes aware of the act, he or she can terminate the act. For example, If you have ever been at a basketball game, you may have observed some spectators throwing imaginary basketballs at strategic moments during the game. Or perhaps you have experienced this while watching a baseball game. You may find yourself throwing a baseball or performing some act you would like to see occur. You may then become aware of what you are doing, feel it is silly and stop performing the act. Another example of nonvoluntary behavior, that almost all motorists have experienced, is while sitting in the passenger's seat, something occurs that demands the automobile be braked immediately. Often the passenger will start pressing on an imaginary break. Once they become aware of what they are doing and realize that it serves no useful purpose, they stop the action. Sometime, if they feel the situation is very dangerous, they find it difficult to stop pushing on the imaginary brake, even though they know it will not help the situation.

Nonvoluntary behavior occurs when we want some action (by us or others) to occur and then find ourselves subconsciously carrying out the act. Usually once we become aware of what we are doing we can terminate the act. There is no sense of willing the act to take place on our part. Probably everyone has at one time or another caught himself unintentionally performing some action that he is watching someone else perform. For example, when we watch someone trying very hard to reach

10

something, we unconsciously tend to reach. This type of behavior tends to occur when our attention is focused on one thing. That is, our mind is occupied by a single dominant thought. Our field of attention is restricted to a single event. This type of behavior is sometimes referred to as ideomotor action.

By **involuntary behavior** we mean some action that an individual performs that he does not initiate, and has no control over. For example, if some object is rapidly approaching your eyes, you will blink. You have no choice. If you touch something very hot with your hand, your hand will immediately remove itself. Again you have no control over the action. If a light is shined in your eye, the pupil of your eye will contract; it is not under your voluntary control. Such behavior is usually due to an inborn reflex. You do not initiate it and you cannot control it.

By **hypnotic behavior** we mean actions that an individual performs in response to suggestions made by a hypnotist. These actions are carried out without any sense of voluntary action on the part of the subject. The subject observes these actions as responses to suggestion that he or she did not initiate. The individual acts in a passive manner; there is no sense of initiating or inhibiting the action. The individual is aware of what is happening and has no desire to control the action. For example, if it is suggested that an individual's hand is becoming very light and will begin to float in the air like a gas filled balloon. To the disbelief of many subjects, this is what occurs. If it should be suggested that the temperature in the room is rapidly dropping below zero. The subject will respond by shivering and goose bumps will appear on his skin. People in the "hypnotic state" tend to react to the suggestions of the hypnotist as though they were reality. If a hypnotist should suggest to a subject that there is a purple alligator in front of him, he will see the alligator, even though he knows he is responding to a suggestion, the alligator is not real and is a hallucination.

From an introspective point of view, the most characteristic difference between actions performed through the influence of suggestion and ordinary acts is that ordinary acts are felt to be willed, while suggested acts are felt not to be willed.

It is probable that any phenomenon which can be produced by suggestion while in the "hypnotic state," can be produced to a lesser degree by suggestions given in the normal waking condition. All observable behaviors described above are actually carried out by the musculature of the individual, which is under the control of his brain and nervous system.

Suggestions are ideational stimuli. They are used to convey an idea from one individual (the hypnotist) to another (the subject) with the intent of soliciting certain responses. These responses do not involve any conscious volitional effort and are neither innate nor acquired adequate responses to the stimulus. A distinguishing characteristic of suggestion is that the response elicited by it is **non**voluntary in its initiation. It never involves the active, conscious, volitional participation of the subject. This does not mean that the subject cannot evaluate or control the response if he wanted to; however, usually he has no desire to do so. The response is behavior in which he is a passive participant. This is why we call it "nonvoluntary" and not "involuntary" behavior.

Behavior as a Continuum

There is no hard-and-fast distinction between our classifications of behavior. In fact they seem to form a continuum in which separating them into categories is arbitrary. The extremes of the continuum manifest very clear differences, but they are a matter of degree.

One phenomena of hypnosis that is very impressive is, suggested behavior that is not considered under voluntary control, can be evoked when a person is hypnotized. We will see later that many involuntary behaviors can be through a process called conditioning, elicited without hypnosis. We can learn to control involuntary behavior.

MODULE 2 - INTRODUCTION TO HYPNOSIS

This is module two in a series of modules about hetero-hypnosis. We will attempt to give a working definition of hypnotism, what it is, hypnotic techniques and methods of inducing the hypnotic trance. In modern hypnosis, suggestion plays a large part in inducing hypnosis.

Nature of Suggestion

Suggestions play a central role in the use of hypnosis and in its induction. Most suggestions are of a verbal nature. They are first of all an ideational stimulus. They are used to convey an idea from one individual to another with the objective of evoking specific responses. The person giving the suggestions is called the *hypnotist* (also suggester or operator). The recipient is called the *subject* (sometimes the suggestee). The responses to these suggestions do not involve any conscious volitional effort on the part of the subject to carry out the suggestions. The responses are of a nonvoluntary nature. When inducing hypnosis or while a subject is in a trance, the hypnotist will sometimes give the subject instructions. For example, the hypnotist may say to the subject, "Stiffen your arm." When the subject does this, it may be that he is just following instructions, or the response may be a reflex-like action. It is difficult to tell and the subject himself may not know. In actual practice, the term "suggestion" is used in a very broad sense, which includes a combination of suggestions proper, and instructions of a nonsuggestive nature.

Responses to Suggestions

When hypnotized, the responses to suggestions by subjects will vary dramatically. Usually the suggestions given by the hypnotist are to the effect that the subjects will have certain experiences or carry out certain acts. Some individuals will not respond at all to any of the suggestions. They feel no compulsion to carry out the suggestions and have no suggested experiences. Such persons are said to be *nonsuggestible*. At the other extreme are people that respond fully to all or some of the suggestions. They are said to be *suggestible*. The suggestible group can be put into two classes. Both classes will tend to lose all awareness of themselves and their surroundings and experience what is being suggested in a very vivid way. One class will respond in an overt way, physically carrying out the suggested activity. For example, if it is suggested that they are digging a hole, they will go all through the actual motions of removing soil with an imaginary shovel. The other class will have the same experience, but will show no physical sign of it. In other words, every aspect of the suggestion is hallucinated but kept at a sensory level.

Most individuals that feel they were not influenced by suggestions and as a matter of fact show no sign of responding will say so. However, some individuals who do not feel they are responding to suggestion will not say anything but will "act out" the suggestions and instructions of the hypnotist as if they were responding. Usually with such people the suggestions do have some effect. They feel a strong compulsion to carry out the suggestions.

It should be pointed out that suggestions are effective to some degree in the waking state. Everyone with out exception (that is willing and cooperative) can be made to demonstrably respond to waking suggestions. This is usually referred to as *ideomotor action.* We will have much more to say about this later.

The State of Hypnosis

Hypnosis is a state of heightened suggestibility usually brought about in an individual by the use of a combination of the visual fixation upon a small object and suggestions of relaxation. There are many different ways and techniques that can be used to produce the hypnotic state. Some are very slow, taking ten to twenty minutes, while others are very rapid, taking only a few seconds. We will cover these in a later module.

As a rule the suggestions or procedures used to produce hypnosis are called *trance-inducing* suggestions or procedures. It is customary to use the word "trance" to describe the hypnotic state. The state of not being hypnotized is referred to as the "waking" state. Because "trance" and "waking" are polar terms, it would suggest that if a person was not in the waking state, he is asleep. This is not the case; a hypnotized person is not asleep.

Extensive experiments have demonstrated that there are no differences between the physiology of the waking state and the hypnotic trance. The electric potentials of the brain are the same. The circulation of blood through the brain is the same. Respiration and the consumption of oxygen are the same. Blood pressure, blood count, heartbeat, and blood analysis are the same.

There are various degrees of the hypnotic state. A subject is said to be in a *light* state of hypnosis when he becomes slightly more hypersuggestible and in a *deep* state when very hypersuggestible. A subject very deep in hypnosis is said to be in a *"somnambulistic state."*

Conditions for Hypnosis

For our purposes we will investigate four basic methods of inducing a state of hypnosis. They are: the Braid method, the Classical method, the Standard method (also known as the Modern method) and the Sensorimotor method.

Over a long period of time people that have investigated and practiced hypnosis have come to the conclusion that certain conditions and procedures are capable of producing the effect.

13

1. **Fixation (or Concentration of attention**
2. **Monotony**
3. **Restricting voluntary movements**
4. **Narrowing the field of consciousness**
5. **Neural Inhibition**
6. Successive response to suggestions

The first of these conditions is specific to the Braid method. The first five are used in the Classical method. The Classical induction method places the subject in an environment structured to utilize one or more of the first five conditions. The Standard method makes use of all six conditions, with the sixth playing a dominant role. The Standard method is sometimes referred to as the Suggestion method. The use of condition six alone constitutes the Sensorimotor method. The Standard method is the most frequently used.

The Standard Method

This method will be described in more detail in another module, but the general process will be presented here. Typically the subject is asked to focus his attention, by fixating on a bright object. As he does this he is presented with suggestions that tend to bring about closure of the eyelids, relaxation and conditions that are similar to natural sleep. This method initially depends upon some degree of waking suggestibility. The more responsive the subject is to waking suggestion, the more rapid the induction will be. The suggestibility of an individual depends upon **three elements: Ideomotor, Semantic conditioning and dissociation.**

Normally a person that has never been hypnotized or submitted to suggestion will only manifest the ideomotor element. If the other elements are present they are usually relatively inactive. The induction of hypnosis consists only of activating the other two elements, or at least conditions that favor their manifestation.

The ideomotor element is called *ideomotor action*. This is the tendency of thoughts or ideas to be automatically translated, reflex-like, into specific patterns of muscular activity appropriate to the thought or idea held by the individual. For example, if an individual thinks about tying his shoelaces, the muscles that would be used to perform that task will be activated to some degree and carry out the task in an aborted way. This is true of every normal individual; it is a reflex that only differs from other reflexes in that it is elicited directly by higher nerve center activity rather than by afferent peripheral impulses. Probably waking suggestions act purely through ideomotor action. An important characteristic of ideomotor action is that as it is repeatedly elicited, it tends to produce a stronger response. This is probably the main reason suggestions are repeated over and over.

When an individual is made to respond to a number of suggestions, there is an increased tendency for him to respond to other suggestions. This is thought to be due to Semantic conditioning. Semantic conditioning occurs when a person carries out an act or has an experience when another person makes

14

a statement describing the act or experience and the two events are closely juxtaposed in time. At such a time there is created, by way of a conditioning process, a tendency for the first person to reflexively exhibit motor and sensory responses associated with the ideational content of the others statements. We will have much more to say about Semantic conditioning in later modules.

The third element of hypnotic suggestibility, *dissociation of awareness,* is necessary for deep hypnosis. In essence it is a selective constriction of awareness that eliminates all sources of stimuli except the suggestions of the hypnotist.

The finial result of any trance induction depends largely upon the degree to which the three elements, ideomotor, Semantic conditioning and dissociation are activated. Some subjects may develop each to a high degree; others may never go beyond heightened ideoaction, while some may only display weak ideomotor action. In addition to the basic elements, there are a number of other factors that can definitely influence the production of hypnosis. They include the attitude, experiences, needs, fears and defenses of the subject. These factors can be altered within limits in order to enhance the subject's ability to enter the hypnotic state.

What we have described so far is primarily concerned with inducing hypnosis using the Standard method. This assumes that the subject initially only shows a capacity for ideomotor action. However, some subjects will also display a certain amount of generalized suggestibility and/or a high capacity for dissociation of awareness. With such subjects a much briefer technique can be used to induce hypnosis.

In summary, the Standard method of inducing hypnosis consists of a combination of sensory fixation and sleep suggestions that activate three processes, ideomotor action, Semantic conditioning, and dissociation of awareness. The dissociation of awareness is developed largely by concentrating the subject's attention upon a fixation object, the suggestions and the hypnotist. Also the attitude, beliefs and expectancies of the subject can help or hinder the induction.

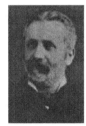

The Braid and Classical Methods

So far we have only discussed the Standard method of inducing hypnosis. We will now turn our attention to the Braid and Classical methods. The Sensorimotor method will be discussed in a later module.

James Braid found that visual fixation on a small bright object by a subject was all that was necessary to induce the so-called mesmeric trance, now called hypnosis. Braid eventually decided that it was not the visual fixation but the concentration of attention that produced the hypnosis. He found that hypnosis could be induced by using any method of focusing the subject's attention. He found that auditory and tactile methods of focusing the attention worked just as well.

15

Bernhiem

In later years (under the influence of Bernheim) it was decided that concentration of attention was directly responsible for hypnosis. It was assumed that suggestion was the key to hypnosis. Because people at that time believed that hypnosis could be induced by fixation, the practice of using this method acted as a suggestion that produced the desire result. Since sensory fixation leads to mental and sensory fatigue, this predisposes the subject to feeling tired and sleepy. When "sleep" is subtly suggested it usually ensues. We will go into the Braid method in greater detail in later modules.

There is little question today that hypnotic, or at least hypnotic-like, phenomena can be induced without going through the typical induction procedures. The Sensorimotor method is proof of this. There is an abundance of evident that shows it is possible to start with simple waking suggestions, proceed to more complex ones and without ever saying a word about sleep, relaxation or anything else usually associated with the induction of a trance state, produce a state of deep hypnosis. The subject will gradually pass from the waking state into hypnosis with no clear transition evident.

MODULE 3 - CONDITIONING AND LANGUAGE

CLASSICAL CONDITIONING

In order to better understand what hypnosis is and why subjects respond to suggestions as they do, we will have to look at how our nervous system works and how we learn to respond to the world around us. All of the information about the world around us is provided by receptors on the surface of our bodies. These receptors are our sense organs -- eyes, ears, nose, skin, tongue, etc. Each of these receptors is connected to your Central Nervous System (CNS) by neurons (nerve cells). There are other nerve cells that go from your CNS (Brain and Spinal Cord) to the muscles and glands of your body. These are called effectors; they affect your muscles and glands in some way. The things in your environment that affect you are called signals. A signal causes a change in one or more of your receptors. A change in your receptor is called the stimulus.

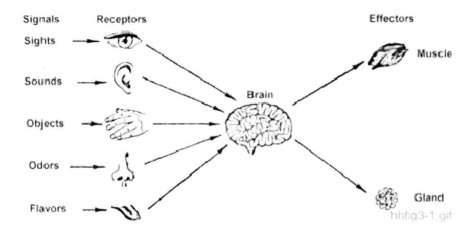

There are many environmental events (signals) going on around us that elicit a response from us. Most of the stimuli we encounter cause us to respond in a predictable manner. For example, loud sounds, electric shock, hot objects, food, visual stimuli, and so on will elicit such responses as the flow of gastric juices, the volume of blood in internal organs, the rate of the heart beat, the blood pressure, the size of the pupil of the eye, activity of the sweat glands and so on. Many of the responses are called reflexes. For example, if you put a piece of candy in your mouth, it will result in the flow of saliva in the mouth. The candy (the signal) stimulates the taste buds that start a nerve impulse that goes to various centers in the CNS, which in turn sends a nerve impulse to the salivary glands that causes them to secrete saliva (the response).

This stimulus-response action is the foundation of all your behavior. Everything you do is a matter of stimulus and response. For example, if you hear some one call your name, you turn to see who is calling. This is what occurs, the sound of your name (the signal) causes a change (the stimulus) in your ear. The change (the stimulus) sends a nerve impulse to a center in your brain that in turn sends a nerve impulse to your muscles. Your muscles then turn you toward the sound. The turning is the response.

The circuit from the receptor (ear, eye, nose, etc.) through the Central Nervous System (brain and spinal cord) to the effectors (muscles or glands) is called the stimulus-response *arc*. This is the mechanism responsible for all human behavior. When a child is first born, his entire behavior is determined by these arcs. The child's behavior is entirely of a reflex nature. However, as the child grows older, he learns to modify, inhibit, enhance and voluntarily control some of these stimulus-response arcs.

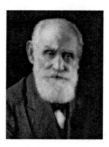

I.P.Pavlov

How we learn to control and modify some of our stimulus-response arcs was first demonstrated by Pavlov. He used dogs to investigate how the S-R arcs function. The same laws apply to human beings, but people seem to object to being experimented on, which is why he used dogs. His fundamental experiments with dogs are well established. We will not go into a detailed account of his experiments here[1].

He demonstrated that signals that did not have the power to elicit a specific response, could gain that power. For example, if a dog is given a piece of meat, the salivary glands secrete saliva. The meat stimulates the flow of saliva. If a bell is rung or a light is turned on, but no meat is given to the dog it did not salivate. Pavlov demonstrated that the ringing of a bell or the turning on of a light could gain the power to make the dog salivate. If a stimulus that does not elicit the salivary response (i.e., the sound of a bell) is paired with the meat, this stimulus will after a number of pairings gain the power to elicit the salivary response. Once the conditioning has occurred, the ringing of the bell alone will elicit the salivary reflex.

The stimulus that originally elicits a response is called the *Unconditioned Stimulus* (US). In the above example, this is the meat. The stimulus that at first does not elicit the response is called the *Conditioned Stimulus* (CS). In our example this is the sound of a bell. If after the conditioning, the CS is presented many times without the US, the response to the CS will begin to weaken. This is known as extinction. However, the response to the CS can be maintained if it is only intermittently paired with the US and can become very resistant to extinction.

Pavlov found salivation could be conditioned to any neutral stimulus that the dog could detect -- sounds of metronomes, buzzers, lights, touches of the finger, etc. One dog was conditioned to salivate when it received an electric shock. At first the shock was very weak so as to be barely perceptible. As the shock was increased in strength it was found that a very strong shock produced no sign of pain or displeasure. There was no quickening of the heartbeat or breathing which usually accompanies an unpleasant event. Instead the shock was followed by mouth-watering and tail wagging.

More recently, J.P. Segundo, at the Instituto de investigacion de ciencias biologicas, in Montevideo, has reported experiments similar to Pavlov's, removal by conditioning, of the sensation of pain from noxious stimuli. In his experiments, cats were conditioned to "turn off" the sensation of pain associated with an electrical shock. In his conditioning procedure, a musical note was sounded a few seconds after the electric current producing the pain was turned off. Eventually, the sounding of the musical note alone would cause the cats to exhibit all the symptoms of relaxation that accompanied the cessation of the painful electric shock even though the current had not been turned off.

It is well known that there is some kind of "switch" in the nervous system that is capable, under certain circumstances, of turning off the sense of pain. Many people have had the experience of being severely injured in a highly excited situation and not be aware of pain until the after the excitement had subsided. This is common among people injured in battle or in automobile accidents.

Some of the most interesting examples of conditioning, where connections between simple stimuli and bodily responses normally not under voluntary control have been conditioned, are found in experiments on humans. In an experiment performed by C.V. Hudgins, the conditioned stimulus was the sound of a bell. The bell was rung and then a light was directed into the eye of the subject. When the light struck the eye the pupil of the eye contracted. This is due to the normal pupillary-control reflex. After many repetitions of this procedure, the sound of the bell alone caused the pupil to contract. Next Hudgins replaced the sound of the bell with the spoken word "contract." In several hours of training, the sound of the word "contract" gained the power to force an involuntary contraction of the pupil.

This is an important discovery. Hudgins, by just saying the word "contract" could now produce a strong contraction of the subject's pupil. This conditioning, with and without retraining, lasted fifteen to ninety days.

Some of his subjects were taught to say the word "contract" aloud as they went through the conditioning procedure. Before long, these subjects could make their pupil contract by saying the word "contract" with out the light or the bell. Later, he conditioned five subjects to contract their pupils when they just *thought* the word "contract." The light or bell was no longer needed. By way of conditioning it was possible to gain control over that which is normally uncontrollable. Other subjects were conditioned to dilate their pupils by thinking the word "relax."

R. Menzies reported an experiment he performed in the *Journal of Experimental Psychology*, 1941. He put a stencil patterned "XX" in front of a blue electric bulb. When the XX pattern was illuminated, he instructed subjects to whisper the word "crosses" while looking at them. Two seconds latter the right hands of the subjects were immersed in ice water. The combination of light and cold continued for about thirty seconds.

It is a neurological fact that if one hand is suddenly chilled, the other will become somewhat chilled also. This is believed to be do to a bilateral reflex action. To the dry left hand a sensitive temperature-recording device was attached. Menzies recorded the drop in temperature of the dry hand as the other was chilled. He conditioned this chilling to the combined stimulus of a blue light and repetition of the word "crosses."

After forty, three minute training sessions, all of the subjects he conditioned upon looking at the light and saying the word "crosses" (without any ice water) produced a measurable drop in temperature of the left hand. The drop in temperature was do to a constriction of blood vessels in the hands. This physical change was produced by a conditioned response to a light-vocal "bell."

Pavlov found that once a stimulus (i.e., Bell) has gained the power to trigger a response (i.e., Salivation) the stimulus can then "pass" the response on to a new stimulus (i.e., A Light). The third stimulus can then elicit a response without ever having been paired with the original environmental stimulus that elicits the response.

Semantic Conditioning

In humans, the meaning of words, can and do act as conditioned stimuli that can produce involuntary bodily functions. For example, if a subject has been conditioned to decrease the diameter of his pupil at the ringing of a bell, the word "ringing" can also produce the same response without the actual ringing of the bell. This will only work with humans, not with other animals. It is not the sound of the word humans react to, but the meaning of the word. On the other hand, if a subject is conditioned to respond to a word, and the stimulus object the word "denotes" is later presented to the subject, the object (never conditioned to elicit the response) will also elicit the response. That is the two stimuli (the word stimulus and the object stimulus) are functionally equivalent.

As an example, lets say the word "red" has been used as the conditioned stimulus in a classical conditioning procedure. It is paired with an electrical shock as the stimulus. After a few trials the word "red" will elicit a conditioned heart response. At a later time if the subject is shown a red light it will be found that the red light will also elicit the conditioned heart response.

The principle underlying classical conditioning is this: If the stimulation of a specific pattern of sensory neurons (nerve cells) in the brain is followed by a specific pattern of activity of motor or glandular neurons, repetition of the sequence will ultimately create neuronal connections so that the sensory pattern alone can directly drive the motor or glandular response. This is an automatic process; it does not involve any consciousness of the procedure. A conditioned reflex, once created, requires no conscious effort. It just happens.

We will mention one more experiment performed by D. G. Ellson. He sat his subjects in a comfortable chair. On the left arm of the chair was a small light bulb. He sounded a thousand cycle tone for several seconds after which the light bulb was illuminated. The tone acting as the unconditioned stimulus was paired with the light acting as the conditioned stimulus. Thirty-two of forty subjects conditioned this way, reported hearing the tone when only the light was presented alone. This means that thirty-two of the subjects were conditioned into hearing auditory hallucinations. In other word, eighty percent of the subjects could not tell the difference between a "real" sound and their own hallucinations.

Human beings are constantly conditioned to words throughout their life. Not to the sound of the word, but to the meaning of the word. Words are the "bells" of conditioned reflexes. Lets see how a child might be conditioned to the concept of an apple. Suppose we show a child a shiny red apple. As we do we say the word "ap-ple." After we do this a few times a neural pattern is created in the child's brain representing the concept of "apple." This pattern would have two components, one auditory one visual. Ultimately the sight of the apple alone would be enough to trigger both the auditory and visual concept of "apple." The spoken word alone would trigger the visual image in the child's imagination of the physical apple. Suppose now we let the child touch the apple each time we show him an apple. The neural pattern in the brain begins to build as the concept of "apple" includes more sensory modalities. Next, we let the child taste and smell the apple. If the child likes the apple, a neural pattern for "pleasure" is created. Next the child may be taught to say the word "apple" as he sees, feels, smells and eats it. When the child has developed the concept apple, The aroma from a near by apple orchard is enough to cause the child to "think" apple. In this case, the odor component triggers the neural pattern that represents the concept apple. When words are conditioned to concepts they become signals, the thinking or speaking of which can elicit the entire package of properties that make up the concept.

Words are the "bells" of conditioned reflexes. Such words as "wonderful," "marvelous," and "beautiful," make us feel good because we have been conditioned to respond to them in that way. The words "freezing," "ice" and "snow" have a cold quality because of their past associations.

What do you see when a good subject is hypnotized? The hypnotist says, "your eyes are so *heavy*, your body feels so tired. You feel so sleepy. You just want to *sleep*. Your body feels *heavy*. Your arms are so *tired*. " And so on. Soon the subject's eyes close and he drifts off into a trance. Is it not plausible that the use of the word "heavy" in good subjects is associated with heavy feeling and the repetitious use of the word acts as a "bell" that triggers actual heavy feelings.

Within the conditioned reflex is the essence of hypnosis. When a hypnotized subject shivers when the hypnotist suggests ice and snow, it is do to verbally conditioned "bells" waiting to be rung. Hypnosis is the eliciting of reactions in a human being through the use of verbal or associated reflexes.

Pavlov refer to the conditioned reflex approach to hypnosis when he said "Speech, on account of the whole preceding life of the adult, is connected up with all the internal and external stimuli which can reach the cortex, signaling all of them and replacing all of them, and therefore it can call forth all those reactions of the organism themselves. We can, therefore, regard 'suggestion' as the most simple form of a typical conditioned reflex in man."

V. M. Bechterev also alluded to the reflex aspect of hypnosis[2]. "Every word, being a sign, is in accordance with the associated-reflex scheme, associated as a secondary stimulus either with an external or internal stimulus, or with some state, posture, or movement of the individual in question. The word consequently plays the role of an external stimulus, and becomes a substitute, according to the association established, for an external influence or a certain inner state."

Language and Thought

Words describe things and events. Everything tends to be given a name (a sound symbol) that permits them to be easily evoked in their absence. However, the word becomes detached from the object or event it signifies and acquires an independent life. From this point on, language is no longer a means of communication, a series of signals between two persons, but an instrument of thought. Only man makes use of an internal language, which is no longer speech, since it is not expressed in sound, but a method of thinking. A word is not some mysterious substance stored in a nerve cell but the functional relationship that exists between millions of neurons.

Although on a physiological plane, language does not differ from other conditioned reflexes, it is a very particular aspect of conditioning, one that only exists in man. Language was considered by Pavlov and his followers as a *secondary system of signals*. The primary system, the system of non-verbal signals, is the only one that exists in animals. Pavlov wrote "As regards man, speech is clearly a conditioned stimulus as real as all those that he has in common with animals, but on the other hand, it goes farther than they go and like no other stimulus, it embraces a multitude of purposes. In this connection, speech allows no comparison, either qualitative or quantitative, with the conditioned stimuli of animals." Later he went on to say "If our sensations and our observations as regards the world about us constitute for us the first signals of reality, the concrete signals, it is speech and, above all, the kinesthetic stimuli (muscular sensitivity) linking the speech organs with the cortex that constitutes the secondary signals, the signals that devolve from signals. They represent an abstraction of reality and lend themselves to a superior generalization, which is exactly what constitutes our specifically human method of thought."

A dog can be trained to react to the word "bell," but the actual ringing of a bell would not produce the same response. The word for the dog has no value except as a signal it has been trained to respond to. It has no general abstract significance that enables it to replace it by the sound of a bell. On the other hand, a human trained to react to a bell can react in the same way to the word "bell" or a synonym of it. The word is a signal of a signal. In the course of a man's development everything that occurs in the primary system of signals acquires a reflex in the secondary system that is always more complete and precise. In man the secondary system predominates over the primary. However, since its acquisition is more recent it is also more fragile. It is the first to disappear in hypnotic states.

1. Pavlov, I.P. Conditioned Reflexes. Oxford University Press, 1927 *Lectures on Conditioned Reflexes.* Vol. I, International Publishers, N.Y., 1928 *Conditioned Reflexes and Psychiatry.* International Publishers, N.Y., 1941

2. Bechterev, V. M. *General Principles of Human Reflexology.* International Publishers, N.Y.

MODULE 4 - MIND SET

DEVELOPING MIND SET

To a majority of people, the word "hypnotism" brings to mind visions of the mysterious. It conveys a suggestion of the supernatural, occultism and the mystical. Most people have a mental image of a "hypnotist" as a tall, dark sinister person with glittering and piercing eyes. Visions of the fictional Svengali or the real-life Rasputin appear in their imaginations. Almost any well-educated intelligent person, the scientist, college professor, business executive, when asked to become a hypnotic subject, shows alarm and quickly declines. They are fearful of damage to their mind or of finding themselves under the power of the hypnotist.

If asked about their knowledge of hypnosis, most would freely admit to a complete lack of knowledge of the subject. Perhaps some have seen a stage demonstration, where people from the audience were placed in a hypnotic state and caused to perform various amusing stunts. The observers leave such stage shows with a feeling of having witnessed weird phenomena, with no inclination for a closer personal experience with such a mysterious power.

In most instances the above misconceptions of hypnosis will not help you as a hypnotist induce a state of hypnosis. In fact they can severely handicap you. We are under the opinion that any "normal" person that is willing and able to follow the instructions of the hypnotist can develop the so-called state of hypnosis. This is something that the subject must do. He and only he can develop a hypnotic trance. You as the hypnotist can only guide him into the hypnotic state. You can help your subject by taking the mystery out of hypnotism. Explain to him that there is nothing mysterious about hypnotism. Most hypnotic phenomena can be explained by known physiological facts.

Usually it is difficult to get most of us to admit it, but many of our beliefs and attitudes are based on erroneous assumptions. We often feel if we see something, or experience it ourselves, we can accept it as a fact. However, when our conclusions are based upon our own experience, without knowledge of scientific methods, we can be wrong.

It is easy to demonstrate how unrealistic we are being when we attempt to rely upon our own perceptions. We will give several examples illustrating this because belief and skepticism are important factors in the success or failure in the development of the hypnotic state. An understanding of the facts and fallacies we derive from our perceptions and beliefs will help alter existing erroneous ideas. We will also explain the physiology behind some hypnotic phenomena.

Retinal Fatigue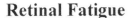

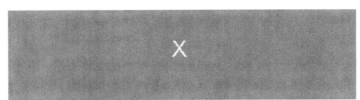

We will perform a little experiment. Just above this paragraph there is a red rectangle with an "X" in the center. We will use this to demonstrate how our perceptions can change with no awareness on our part. Take a white card or white piece of paper and cover the left or right half of the rectangle. Now stare fixedly at the line formed by the contrasting areas for about 20 seconds. If part of the "X" is visible, you can fix your gaze on that. Keeping your eyes focused on the same area (i.e., part of the "X") remove the white card or paper exposing the rest of the colored area. It will appear that the half of the rectangle that was covered seems to be a brighter color than the exposed half of the rectangle.

Of course, the color has not changed at all; it is the perception of the observer that has changed. The change in perception is only a temporary change, almost immediately the two areas will appear the same. This indicates that another change in perception has occurred.

For a more dramatic demonstration of the same phenomena, do the following. On a blank sheet of white paper, draw a single, horizontal pencil line about two to three inches long. Fix your gaze on the center of the line. As you continue to stare at the line, you will notice that the line begins to appear gray and eventually disappears altogether. The whole phenomena should take approximately 30 seconds. Once you remove your gaze from the area of the paper where the line is and then look again at the area, you will see the pencil line.

To understand what is occurring in our two experiments, you need to know how nerve cells function. The sensation we call sight results from light being reflected from the object we are looking at to our eyes. The image of the object is focused on the retina of the eye the same way an image is focused on the film of a camera.

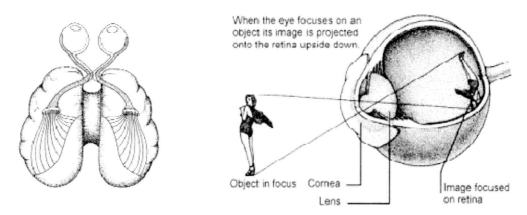

When the eye focuses on an object its image is projected onto the retina upside down.

Object in focus   Cornea
Lens
Image focused on retina

The image focused on the retina of the eye activates receptor cells that start nerve impulses that eventually reach the visual center (occipital Cortex) in the brain. Here a pattern of interconnecting nerve cells (neurons) is created that represent the image focused on. This representation of what we are looking at is inside out head, however, we have learned that it belongs outside of ourselves and project it there.

Now the question remains, why did the color fade and why did the pencil line disappear in our experiments. This is due to the nature of neurons (nerve cells). Neurons operate on the All-or-None principle. They transmit messages at maximum strength or not at all. They transmit impulses like machine gun bullets rather than like the continuous flow of water. There is a refractory period of a nerve fiber that sets the limit at which it can respond to repeated stimulation. Prolonged activity of nerve cells causes them to become fatigued. When this occurs, the rate at which they can be reactivated is prolonged. It is due to the frequency of the neurons "firing" that causes the color to fade in our experiment. Also, the receptor cells in the retina of the eye contain chemical elements that are "used up" as we fix our attention on the red color. The sensation of "red" is diminished, but so gradually that we are unaware of it.

The process illustrated above is called retinal fatigue. It is a principle that has been well confirmed and excepted by all men of science. It illustrates the point that what we think we see is not always truly representative of the facts. In our experiment we have evidence that our perception of color can become altered without our being aware of it. It also shows how quickly nerve cells can be fatigued and fail to function (i.e., the pencil line vanishes). In our examples, only by shifting the gaze or blinking periodically will the chemical elements be replenished and our sight maintain some degree of

Dual Image

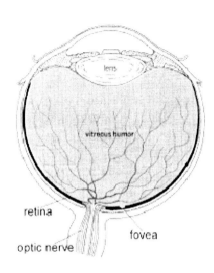

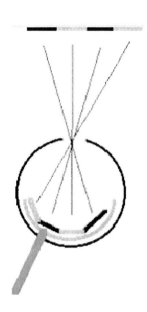

When you look at an object, each of your eyes sees a slightly different view of the object you are focusing on. If you will look at a small three-dimensional object about two to three feet in front of you, you will see an object that is different than the one seen by your left and right eye. That is, what you see is slightly different than what is seen by your eyes.

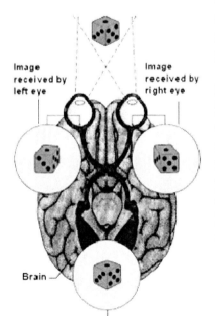

If you will look at some near by object, then close your left eye, the image will slightly change. Try looking at the object with the right eye as you close the left eye, you will see a slightly different view of the object. If you alternately close your left eye as you open your right eye and visa versa, the object will appear to jump to the left as you close the left eye and jump to the right as you close the right eye and open the left. The drawing below illustrates what is occurring. Each eye sees a slightly different view of the same object. Your brain coordinates the two different views into one three dimensional image.

Seeing More Than Your Eye Sees

If you are like most people you assume that what you see is pretty close to what your eye sees. That is the neural pattern created in your brain is pretty faithful to what you are viewing. Not so, your brain adds very substantially to the report it gets from your eyes. A lot of what you see is actually "created" by the brain.

Because of the way the eyeball is constructed it is possible to demonstrate this to yourself. As shown in the illustrations above, the front of the eye acts like a camera lens, which directs light rays from each point in your field of vision onto the retina of the eye. The retina acts something like a sheet of film in a camera. But the retina has a hole in it where the optic nerve exits the eye. At this location there are no receptors that can send information to the brain about what is located in this part of your field of vision. Because of this you have a "blind spot" (one for each eye) near the center of your field of vision where you can't see. See the drawings below. The blind spot is where the optic nerve exits the eye, the red line in the smaller drawing.

Look around and see if you can find the blind spot. Perhaps you can't find it because the blind spot for one eye is at a different place in your field of vision than the blind spot for the other eye (this is true). Therefore, you don't notice it because each eye sees what the other doesn't. Try closing one eye and look around. Still can't find it? Maybe it's so small that you or your brain just ignores it. Not so, actually the blind spot is pretty BIG. You can easily find it if you will look at the drawing below and follow   instructions.

Close your left eye and stare at the cross mark with your right eye. While continuing to focus on the cross mark, you should be able to see the black spot to the right. DO NOT look at it; just be aware of its existence. Slowly move toward the screen as you continue to focus on the cross mark. When you reach a point approximately a foot from the screen the spot will disappear. At this point the light reflected by the spot is falling on an area of the retina where there are no sensors (where the optic nerve exits). What you see in place of the spot is a white field. This is something the brain is making up since the eye is not sending any information about that location in your field of vision. If you continue to move closer to the screen, the spot will reappear.

+   ●

Now lets do a similar experiment on a colored background. Repeat the procedure above using the drawing below. When the spot vanishes, the brain not only matches the background color but also completes the line across the blind spot.

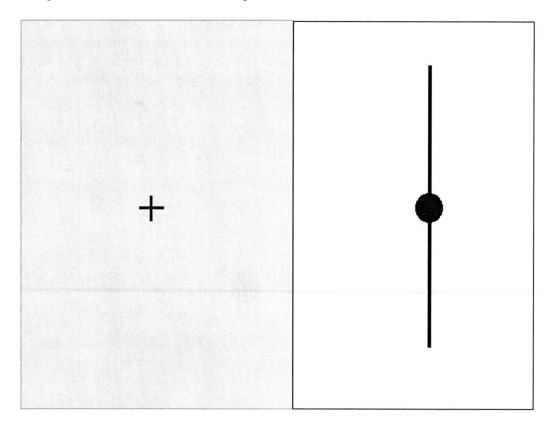

"Free Will"

The ambiguous figure below can be used to demonstrate some interesting observations about the meaning and existence of "free will." Most people will agree that "free will" has two relative distinct properties. One is the idea that what one does is in some sense "free," that is "not determined by something else." The second is the idea that one can oneself control what one does.

Notice that the figure below can sometimes be seen as consisting of dark blue arrows pointing to the right. However, at other times it can be seen as light blue arrows pointing to the left. It is virtually never seen as pointing in both directions at the same time. Whether you see right or left pointing arrows most easily can be influenced by the construction of the figure (i.e., colors, exact shapes, etc.), experiences with other figures, personal preferences, and present mood. However, with all of these held constant, as they are as you look at the figure at this moment, the figure can still be seen in two different ways. In other words, your perception of the figure is a variable in a way that seems "not to be determined by anything else." This implies that if you were to look at the figure a second time you can control what you do. To make this observation, close your eyes and decide if you want to see the

28

arrows pointing to the right or left. Once you have decided, open your eyes and look at the figure. Is the figure pointing in the direction you decided? Try this experiment several times.

If you saw the figure pointing in the direction you had decided on, it means you have taken an action which was not determined by anything else (since the figure could be seen either way) and which you controlled (since you decided which way to see the figure). This suggests that you have a free will (aren't you glad). If you did not immediately see the arrows pointing in the direction you had decided, it indicates that the power of free will does not extend to determining what you see. What you see at any given time is determined by actions of your brain that you cannot fully control. However, since you are able to see the arrows pointing in the direction you decided (although not immediately upon opening your eyes) you are still executing some form of "free will."

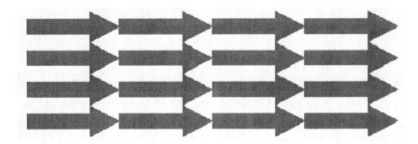

Visual Hallucinations and Dreams

You should understand that when you look at an object (i.e., a red box) you do not really "see" the object itself. You "see" the light reflected by the object to your eye. The lens of your eye forms a picture of the object on the back (the retina) of your eye, just like a camera forms an image on a photographic film. This image starts neural impulses that go to the visual center of your brain. This results in a pattern of interconnecting neurons being formed. It is this neural pattern that represents the object you are looking at (i.e., a red box). The images we see are in our head, we project them out side of ourselves. We have learned by using our other senses that is where the real object is. When you are asleep, the same pattern of interconnected neurons can re-occur. If it should be a pattern that represents a red box, you see the red box in your dream. It seems real, because in a sense it is real. We all have dreams and except them as normal. If a hypnotist should suggest that a subject sees a red box, and the subject does, most people think this is strange. Something mystical is occurring. The hallucinations that are produced while in a state of hypnosis are coming from the same source as dreams. A neural pattern of interconnecting nerve cells that represent the hallucination has been reestablished. Dreams and hallucinations come from the physical interconnections of millions of nerve cells in patterns that represent the images seen in dreams and hallucinations. However, when we dream or are under hypnosis, a logical critical part of our mind is not working. You have learned that you cannot walk through a brick wall, but in your dreams you can and in a state of hypnosis you can, because this logical analytical part of your brain is not active. In childhood we learn that we should not see things, unless there is some stimulus from the world out side of ourselves, that triggers the image. A few people have failed to learn this and see things that are not real; we call them crazy.

Double Vision

When you focus on some near by object, all objects in the distance are doubled and when you focus on a far object all near objects are doubled. Hold the index finger of each hand upright and in line before your eyes, one six inches in front of the nose, the other twelve inches beyond your nose. If you look at the closest finger, the far one is doubled. Now look at the far finger, and you will find that the near one is double. Usually these double images are not seen or are "neglected" if they are dimly perceived. This is an example of how we have learned to control our field of conscious awareness. Ordinarily we have a wide field of conscious awareness that is indefinitely and vaguely bounded. Within this field of awareness we have learned to focus our attention on what is important to us at the moment. This ability to narrow our field of conscious awareness applies to all of our senses, not only sight. In the state of hypnosis the field of attention closely approaches in size and shape the field of conscious awareness. The limitation of the field of awareness is drawn into the limitation of the field of attention.

Varying the Field of Attention

You have learned to easily change your field of attention. For example, you might be standing on a busy city street-corner having a conversation with a friend, while at the same time be aware of an airplane overhead, a passing truck, and a band near by playing a march. You can at will choose to focus your attention on any of the currents events. On the other hand, you may be so engrossed in the conversation with your friend that you may restrict your attention to your conversation to the point that you are unaware to the airplane, truck and band.

Doubt Skepticism and Conviction

I think the above examples will be enough to convince you that reactions can be affected and controlled to a predictable degree upon applying the proper methods for doing so. Belief can be changed to doubt. Skepticism and doubt can be replaced with belief. Belief can be increased to conviction.

Most of us have a degree of skepticism about things that are not familiar. The "unknown" often evokes some amount of doubt or apprehension. Feelings such as these can be the basis of resistance. Resistance to accept changes of existing conditions, changes to established beliefs, and to act in a manner contrary to the dictates of our perceptions; even after we recognize our perceptions are wrong.

When you work with a potential subject, a belief in the methods you will use will be a major factor. Skepticism must be brought to at least a neutral level. The way to inhibit any resistance to hypnosis will be to have your subject perform a series of experiments we will present. If you are learning hypnosis, it would be a good idea for you to perform the experiments on yourself. If you have a helper, you might take turns performing the experiments on each other. If you have a belief and confidence in the methods you use, so will your subject.

A series of experiments will be presented in module five of this series. Each will be explained as it is presented and each will be a little more complex than the preceding one. As you practice each succeeding experiment your belief in yourself and in your ability to utilize these techniques will increase. You can use these experiments to reduce the skepticism of potential subjects. As you and/or your subject become more and more familiar with the phenomena observed, which will increasingly be related to hypnosis, apprehension of the unknown will disappear.

MODULE 5 -- WAKING SUGGESTIONS

Ideomotor Action

There are many hypnotic techniques that depend on leading the subject (directly or by inference) to believe that there is a power or force involved in the process of producing hypnosis. This is not our intention. We do not want to develop any false beliefs. In fact we hope to remove even the smallest shred of implication that may connect these techniques with any mysterious, supernatural power or force. We hope to establish a firm belief in the scientific basis of these techniques.

In the experiments that follow, the responses are evoked by ideas and images in the mind of the subject. These ideas and images create impulses in the brain that trigger muscular activity appropriate to the idea of action in the individual's thought processes. This muscular activity is initially very weak. It is only a small fraction of the activity that would result if the subject were to actually perform the full movement instead of just imagining he is doing so.

It has been demonstrated many times using delicate electronic instruments that when a person thinks about performing a physical act (i.e., tying a knot), the muscles that would be used to actually perform the action become energized. The movements are small and are difficult to observe with the naked eye, but they always exist. This is true for every normal human being. If you think about playing a piano, there will be muscular activity affecting the fingers generated. You have no control over this phenomenon it just happens.

In the experiments that follow, the presence of another pattern of strong muscular action or tension involving the same muscles or part of them will mask or block the weak pattern induced by thoughts. For this reason, a certain amount of relaxation seems to favor ideomotor action. However, too much relaxation can be counter productive. A certain amount of general muscle tonus is desirable for optimal effect. Deep relaxation produces an active inhibitory effect, which serves as a blocking agent in respect to muscular activity.

Chevreul's Pendulum

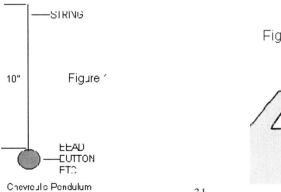

STRING

10"

Figure 1

LEAD
CUTTON
ETC.

Chevreul's Pendulum

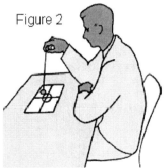

Figure 2

31

This is one of the oldest demonstrations of suggestibility, but a very enlightening one. Chevreul, in 1812, was the first to recognize the nature of the phenomenon involved. It is of interest because it is one of the simplest experiments to perform. Despite its simplicity, it can be used to demonstrate several of the properties of suggestibility. It can also be used to get an indication of an individual's susceptibility to hypnosis.

Before you attempt to use this experiment, you should read the entire demonstration. There are many ways of performing this experiment, and later on when you are more familiar with it, you can use your own version of it. If you are just learning hypnosis, you should try the experiment on yourself. If you have a helper, try the experiment on each other.

First you have to make a pendulum. This is nothing but a small weight hanging on a thread or string. If you want to be more professional, use a light chain instead of string. You can probably buy a pendulum at a magic shop; most have intriguing pendulums made from crystal, plastic, glass or onyx. Some may have "magic" potions or exotic substances embedded in the spheres. However, your homemade one will work just as well. You can use a spherical button about ½ inch in diameter tied to the end of an ordinary piece of thread about 10 inches long. See Figure 1. Actually the color and shape are unimportant.

You should try this experiment yourself. Sit at a table; rest your forearm (left or right) near the front edge of the table. Rest your other elbow with your arm lifted vertically a little in front of your other arm. Hold the end of the thread attached to your pendulum, between your thumb and first finger. The pendulum should hang in front of the center of your body (medium plane) and the bob should be approximately an inch from the tabletop. See Figure 2. Actually, none of these details are crucial. If you just approximate them, the experiment is almost certain to succeed. In fact, if you don't have a table, you can do the experiment standing up.

Use your free hand to steady the weight so that it comes to a standstill. Now imagine a line on the table running from left to right. As you imagine the line, the pendulum will begin to swing, slightly at first, back and forth along the line. Another variation is to imagine that the pendulum is the pendulum on a grandfather's clock. In your imagination, see it swing from side to side like a pendulum on a clock. Once it starts to swing, it will increase its motion even if you think intermittently of something else, as long as your thoughts do not involve a different motion. See Figure 3.

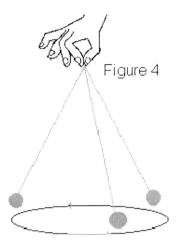

Figure 4

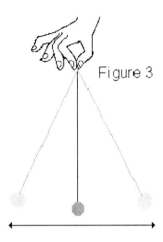

Figure 3

After you have the pendulum swinging for a while imagine that it is swinging on a line going toward and away from you. As you develop this image, the pendulum will slow down and then begin to swing with increasing amplitude back and forth, toward and away from you. After you have done this for awhile, imagine that the pendulum is on the outer edge of a phonograph record and is going around and around in a circle. See Figure 4.

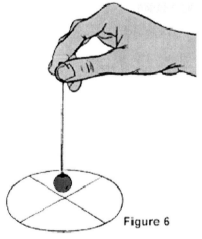

Figure 6

Once you get the pendulum going well in one direction, you can cause it to stop and then revolve in the opposite direction, or just make it stand still. It will obey whatever thought you have in your mind. See Figure 5.

You will probably succeed with the experiment as presented above, very few people fail. If you do not get any positive results, do not give up. Some individuals have to try several times before they can get more than small irregular motions. Try a number of times on consecutive days. Try using different lengths of thread and different bobs, some heaver or lighter. The movement in your fingers is very small. It is the length of the thread that amplifies the motion. In general, the longer the thread the greater the motion.

If you still have difficulty, try drawing a large circle with a cross inside that touches the circle at four points on a piece of paper. See Figure 6 below. Place the paper on the table and try the experiment again. This time start with the pendulum over the intersection of the straight lines and imagine it swinging in the direction of one of the lines. Let your eyes follow along one of the lines as you think of the pendulum following it.

Regardless of the results you have obtained experimenting on yourself, try it using a subject (your helper). Give him the pendulum and have him sit at the table. Instruct him to concentrate on the bob and pay close attention to what you tell him. Then say:

> **Note: The suggestions given here and in the following experiments are intended to be taken only as models. All situations in which suggestions are given tend to be unique in various aspects. You should use your own words, and tailor your suggestions as the situation demands.**

"I would like you to look at the small bob. Fix your attention on it. Don't think of anything but the bob and what I am going to tell you. Let yourself relax and continue to stare at the bob. As you watch the bob you will see that it begins to move a little. In which direction it moves is unimportant. It is going to move, a little at first, then a little more. It is beginning to move a little now, it is beginning to swing. See it is moving a little. Just keep watching it. Think of it as moving. As you do it will move more and more."

> **By this time the bob should be moving. As soon as you can determine the direction it is beginning to move in, suggest that it is moving in that direction. If it seems to be moving in a circular motion, suggest that it is moving in a circle. If it seems to be moving sideways, continue as follows:**

"See, it is moving sideways. It is moving back and forth, back and forth. [If possible, synchronize your voice with the actual motion of the bob.] It is swinging more strongly, back and forth, back and forth. Now you cannot stop the bob from moving. If you try to stop the bob it only makes it move faster, back and forth." [Only give the suggestion that the subject cannot stop the bob, if you are getting a good response.].

Lets stop here and analyze the procedures and suggestions we have used. It is important that you understand the reasons for each step we have asked you to follow. This will help you better relate practice to theory and fact. One obvious application of theory and fact is the request to have the subject fixate on the bob of the pendulum. If this induces any degree of hypnosis, our suggestions will be more effective. In any case, the focusing of attention on the bob will probably tend to prevent stray thoughts from entering the subject's mind, which could compete with those being suggested. If you suggest that the pendulum is going to move, you don't want the subject thinking "He says it is going to move, I wonder if it will really move, I remember seeing a pendulum on a clock moving, I guess I shouldn't be doubting..." Focusing his attention on the bob will tend to prevent these kinds of thoughts from passing through his mind.

The effectiveness of suggestions depends on several factors. There is the subject's innate capacity for ideomotor action or innate suggestibility. Another factor is his attitude. A negative attitude will certainly not help, while a positive one will help. A negative attitude will set up muscular tension patterns that interact with those set up by the suggestions. Abstract conditioning, which is also a part of suggestibility, is relatively sensitive to attitudes. For this reason, proper timing, as well as the proper choice of words is of paramount importance in giving effective suggestions. If you should tell the subject, contrary to facts, that something is occurring or is going to happen, he is likely to form an unfavorably mind set. However, if he experiences events taking place as they are suggested, he tends to form a positive mind set for subsequent suggestions. Therefore, in the Chevreul pendulum experiment you do not want to tell your subject that the bob is moving in a circle if it is in fact moving sideways. If you want the subject to make the bob move in a circle when it is moving sideways, tell him: "The bob is swinging very strongly now. Soon it will begin to change its course and move in a circle. It is going to move in a circle. See, it is beginning to change its motion now. Soon it will move in a circle. There, it is beginning to move in a circle."

You may want to experiment with the way you initially suggest how the pendulum will move. You might start by suggesting it will move in a certain way or direction or you might suggest the pendulum is going to move, but not specify a direction. The main point is to watch what the pendulum is doing and tailor your suggestions accordingly. You want to be sure that the subject experiences what is being suggested. This is a prerequisite for the production of abstract conditioning. If your suggestions contradict what is actually occurring, this conditioning will certainly not take place, and a negative, inhibition-like effect may be induced.

Timing and Proper Wording

Timing and proper wording means, among other things, that when you give suggestions you should alter the model suggestions given in this module to fit various situations you encounter. Subjects tend to react in individual ways. Some will respond very slowly, others very quickly, some will produce motion of large amplitudes, and others will only produce slight motions at the start. You will have to tailor your suggestions accordingly. For example, if there is a large movement of the pendulum immediately after you have suggested movement, then right away say: "See it is moving." If the movement should be sideways, continue by saying that it will be a sideways motion and enhance the motion by saying: "It is moving sideways more and more ... more ... and more ... It is swinging more and more strongly." You may want to change the motion into a circular motion by saying: "It is moving sideways now, but as you continue to focus on the pendulum, the motion will begin to change into a circular one. Soon the bob will begin to rotate ... round ... and round. Think of a circle ... See the motion is changing. It's moving in a circle. The circle is getting larger, the pendulum is moving faster."

Often the pendulum will oscillate and even swing a little from the beginning, even before you have given any suggestions, because the subject's hand is not perfectly steady. Obviously, it would be absurd to tell the subject that the pendulum is going to move when it is already moving. In this situation, impress on the subject that he should relax and not be tense. You can also hold the bob, and keep it still for a moment. If you cannot prevent some initial movement and the subject is aware of it, then call the subjects attention to it in the following way: "You may notice that the bob is moving a little, Don't pay any attention to this, it is because your hand is shaking a little. However, in a few moments you will notice that the bob will move more strongly. You will also notice that it begins to move in a definite direction, perhaps sideways, right and left, or around and around, in a circle ... It will move...See it is already moving a little stronger ... It is definitely getting stronger. Now it is moving from side to side (*or whatever way it is moving*)."

Because you want to time your suggestions properly, you usually should not go to fast in giving your suggestions. If you do, you may tell the subject something is happening before it happens. However, there may be times when there are indications that an event is going to take place. In such cases, you can suggest that it is occurring. Sometimes a suggested event occurs so quickly after the suggestion of its future occurrence that you will have to immediately make a positive statement about its occurrence.

One way you can prevent yourself from getting ahead too fast is to use repetition. Also repetition enhances suggestibility in a cumulative manner. You may find that a subject gives a very weak response to a suggestion, or no apparent response at all. Through repetition alone it is possible build on the suggested idea to the point where a response is clearly detected. Another way repetition helps the effectiveness of suggestions is through monotony. Monotony is believed by many hypnotists to have the ability to bring on the hypnotic state.

The basic idea in this experiment is to get the subject to think of the pendulum as moving without conflicting thoughts occurring. The pendulum will move in response to his thinking and the ease with which it occurs will give you some indication (although not conclusive) of his ability to enter the hypnotic state. Experiment with the pendulum phenomena until you are thoroughly familiar with them, and your subject's responses to them. In module six we will present a number of experiments that operate on the same principle. They represent other demonstrations of psychical control over our physiological responses and will facilitate in developing the hypnotic state.

MODULE 6 - WAKING SUGGESTIONS

Ideomotor Action

The following experiments involve no new principles or factors, but are more steps toward psychical control of physiological responses that will facilitate the development of the hypnotic state. Read the instructions thoroughly so that you completely understand what you are to do. You should try each experiment on yourself and then with a helper. When you practice these experiments it is important

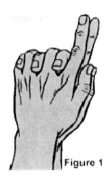

Figure 1

that you have no feeling of urgency. Plan to set aside enough time to complete each experiment with out interruption.

Magnetized Fingers

In order to try this experiment on yourself, sit in a comfortable chair; clasp your hands together. Rest your elbows against your body, and hold your hands about ten inches from your face. Separate your first fingers comfortably as far as possible. Stare at your first fingers for a short time and then close your eyes. See Figure 1.

Now imagine that your fingers are made of steel, and are very strongly magnetized. Imagine that a magnetic force is pulling your fingers together. Imagine that as they are drawn closer together, the magnetic force gets stronger and stronger. Imagine you can feel the magnetic force attracting the fingers together. When you feel the fingers touch, imagine the force is so strong that you cannot separate them. If you have trouble imagining the attraction between your fingers, you might get two small magnets and experiment with them to familiarize yourself with the forces involved.

In this experiment and those following, make up your mind that once you start an experiment, you will concentrate as much as possible on the ideas presented. If other thoughts occur to you, force them aside and return to your original thoughts (i.e., a strong magnetic force). If you find yourself trying to analyze what is actually occurring, use this as a signal to get your mind back on course.

When you use words to make suggestions to yourself, think in terms of the "second" person. Think "you" not "I." Think as though your "conscious" mind were giving orders to your "subconscious mind."

As you perform the experiments, do not be discouraged if you do not get immediate or complete results. Many will be able to get satisfactory results the first time they try performing these experiments, others will require several practice sessions. Your attitude is a major factor in achieving good results. When something occurs in a satisfactory way, you should let the success build your confidence in your ability to use these techniques. Magnify as much as possible your successes and minimize any lack of response in your mind.

A proper degree of cooperation is important. This does not mean you should just go ahead and perform the required responses consciously. It means that you should eliminate any doubt in your mind that a response will occur. Act "as if" the imagined situations were actually reality and as if the responses were actually occurring because of the existing situation.

When you try this experiment with your helper (the subject) you might proceed as follows: Have the subject position his hands as shown in Figure 1. You can have the subject sitting or standing. Grasp the tips of the subject's fingers and tell him that in a moment you will ask him to close his eyes and imagine that his fingers are magnets. Tell him to imagine he can feel a magnetic force pulling his fingers together. As you are giving him these instructions, actually slowly force his fingers together. Now separate his fingers, tell your subject to stare at an imaginary spot between the two fingers. Then

37

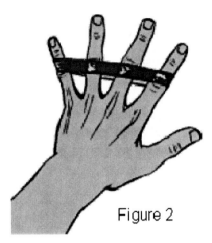

Figure 2

say to him: "As you continue to stare at the imaginary spot I will count from three down to one." "At the count of one, let your eye lids close...three...two...one." "Eye lids close...now tighten your fingers and imagine your first fingers are magnets and that a strong magnet force is pulling them together." "Feel the force getting stronger and stronger." "The more you try to resist the stronger the force gets." "Your fingers are moving...moving...coming closer and closer together." "They are almost touching, the force is getting very strong...very strong." "Open your eyes and look at your fingers."

As pointed out in module five, you may have to alter the model suggestions given above to fit the situation. If you watch the subject's fingers carefully, you will observe that they move in small jerky movements. This is typical of ideomotor responses; the muscular movements tend to occur in small little erratic movements, not in a smooth continuous motion.

Practice the magnet fingers experiment until you feel comfortable with it before going on to the following experiments.

The Rubber Band Experiment

You can try this experiment on yourself in any comfortable position, sitting or lying down. Position one arm in a position where it is easy to keep your eyes focused on the fingers and the back of your hand. See Figure 2 above. With your eyes fixed on your hand, spread your fingers apart as far as possible. Now imagine there is a very strong rubber band stretched around your fingers. Think of the rubber band as a very thick band with a small diameter. See your fingers inserted through the rubber band stretching it as far as possible. Imagine you can feel the rubber band pulling your fingers together. Think to yourself: "The harder you try to keep your fingers apart, the more the rubber band pulls them together. See this occurring in your mind. Now let your eyelids close as you continue to feel the rubber band pulling your fingers together. Imagine that you are trying very hard to keep your fingers apart, but the harder you try the stronger the rubber band becomes. Imagine you can see the rubber band forcing your fingers together, and think the words, the harder you try to keep your fingers apart, the more tired they feel and the more they are drawn together.

Work on this experiment until you get a good response. After your fingers touch, continue to imagine that the rubber band is keeping them very, very tightly together for a short time. Then imagine that the rubber band is gone. Let your fingers relax.

Remember to keep a strong positive attitude while performing this experiment. If you have any difficulty, it probably would help if you actually performed the experiment using a real rubber band. This will help you to actually experience the sensation of real pressure exerted by the rubber band.

Try the experiment with your helper. Tailor your suggestions to him using the procedure outlined above.

The Weight and Balloon

Like the preceding experiments this one involves an ideomotor response. That is the enervation of groups of muscles appropriate to the idea or mental image held by the subject. When you experiment on yourself, it is probably better if you are sitting. When experimenting on your helper, he can be sitting or standing.

Read the following instructions until you are sure you understand them and can proceed without referring to them.

Position yourself in a comfortable chair. Place your feet flat on the floor. You should be able to lean back against some firm support, the back of a chair or a wall. While in this position, extend both arms out straight in front of you at shoulder height with your palms facing one another. See Figure 3. Let your eyelids close. Now, visualize as clearly as possible that a gas filled balloon is tied to your right wrist. It is a big, blue balloon and is pulling at your arm. See it lifting your arm, higher and higher. Develop a clear image of the balloon tugging at your arm, pulling it up higher and higher. See the color of the balloon and its size. Visualize how it is tied to your wrist. Think of your arm floating up, higher and higher.

Once you have the above idea clearly in mind, see a very heavy lead weight tied to your left wrist with a strong rope. Think of how heavy the weight is, visualize its size and shape. Imagine your left arm is so heavy you are unable to hold it up. See it falling lower and lower.

Alternately visualize each of these two concepts for a few seconds. If you find yourself thinking of the actual position of your arms, try to get your mind back to thinking of the balloon and the weight. After two or three minutes, open your eyes. Your hands should be several inches horizontally apart. Your left hand will be lower than your right hand.

Normally if you held your arms in this manner, they would both become heavy and you would find it difficult in maintaining this position more than a few seconds. In this experiment one arm become heavy while the other becomes increasingly lighter. Only a few inches difference indicates success. However, these few inches must occur automatically while you are holding the above concepts in mind, not by just "doing it." When you get satisfactory results from this experiment, try it with your helper. Take turns practicing on each other.

Magnetic Hands

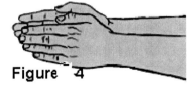

Figure 4

This experiment is similar to the magnetic fingers exercise, except it will involve a larger group of muscles. Although you can practice this experiment on yourself, we will present it as you would practice it with your helper (subject). Have your subject hold his hands as in the weight and balloon experiment. See Figure 4 above. Palms facing palms, but some distance away from each other. Now suggest that a magnetic force is going to pull his hands together. Grasp his hands and slowly move them towards each other. Now separate them and tell your subject to look at an imaginary spot between his two hands. Then say to him. "As you continue to look at the imaginary spot I will count from three down to one." "At the count of one, let your eye lids close and imagine your hands are magnets that are attracting each other. " "Three...two...one, let your eyelids close." "Think of your hands being strongly attracted to each other." "Your hands are beginning to move, coming closer and closer together." "The more you try to resist, the stronger the force pulling then together becomes." "They are moving closer and closer...the closer they come to each other the stronger the force becomes..it is getting very strong now." "Moving closer and closer, they are almost touching now...the force is getting much stronger." "They are moving faster and faster...they are almost touching now...NOW THEY ARE TOUCHING!" "Open your eyes and look at your hands."

Remember, the suggestions given above are only offered as a model. Do not try to memorize any of these models word for word. What you need to learn is the meaning behind the suggestions. You must time your suggestions to fit the current situation. Use your own words to paint a verbal picture that you want to convey to the mind of the subject. You cannot induce hypnosis by memorizing some magic formula that you repeat verbatim. It is the *pattern* and *content* of the suggestions, more than the actual words that are important. The basic idea in the above experiments is to get the subject to think certain thoughts or visualize certain concepts. If you are successful, his own thoughts will automatically be translated, reflex-like, into specific patterns of muscular activity. Ideomotor action is a reflex that only differs from the more common variety in that it is triggered directly by higher center activity rather than by afferent peripheral impulses.

It is very important that your subject does not use his critical faculties to analyze the suggestions you are giving him; especially at the time they initially take effect. It is a good idea to instruct your subject to make his mind blank, to be completely passive, not to think or analyze what is being suggested, or what he is experiencing.

Hand and Arm Levitation Experiment

As you will see in a latter module, this experiment can be turned into a very effective method for inducing hypnosis (i.e., Wolberg's method). There are several ways to carry out this experiment; the following is one of the simpler ones.

Have your subject sit in a chair and place his hand (right or left - subject's choice) on his lap. Now say to him the following:

"Please sit in this chair and position yourself as comfortably as possible...Now just relax and focus your attention on your right (or left) hand." "Think only of your hand and listen to my voice." "As you continue to look at your hand, let yourself become aware of all the sensations occurring in your hand." "In a few moments you may notice a strange feeling in your hand." "You may become aware of a feeling of numbness, or perhaps a tingling sensation." "The kind of sensation doesn't really matter." "Very soon your hand will begin to move." "Just how, I do not know, but it will move." "Maybe a finger will move or maybe just the tip of a finger." "Watch it very carefully, see if you can feels the blood flowing through your hand." Just continue to watch your hand and think of it as moving." "Very

40

shortly you hand is going to move...You feel as if your hand is about to move." "It is moving a little...[*If it moves, add immediately: "There, it is moving some more."*] "Very soon you will feel a sensation of lightness moving into your hand and into your arm." "Think of your hand as being hollow...like as balloon filled with gas." "Your hand is becoming lighter...and lighter, and soon your hand will begin to rise from your lap." "Let the feeling of lightness flow back into your arm." "Your hand and arm will begin to rise from your lap and keep rising because they are becoming so light." It is as though a balloon filled with gas were tied to your hand pulling it up and up into the air." "With every breath you take your hand and arm are becoming lighter...and lighter." You can feel your hand getting lighter and lighter." "It is going to be light as a feather and will float in the air." "There is a force pulling your hand and arm up...up." "Your hand is beginning to rise, your hand is rising." "Your arm is rising." "Your arm and hand are rising...rising...more and more..they are going...up...up...UP!"

If you are successful with this experiment, the subject's hand and arm will rise up in the air. You should question your subject as to the kind of sensations he was having. If he should tell you that he felt a magnetic force pulling his hand and arm up, next time you repeat the experiment with this subject, suggest that he will feel a magnetic force pulling his hand up. Most subjects will report having felt a lightness or that some force was pulling their arm and hand up.

It is quite helpful when giving these suggestions to watch for any kind of motion of the hand or arm and to point them out to the subject. Very often at the beginning a finger will twitch slightly. If this occurs, you should immediately point this out to the subject. You might say: "See, one of your fingers just moved." "Soon this is going to spread...soon your entire hand will move (etc.)." If following these suggestion, other fingers move, remark: "See the movements are spreading, " As soon as you see his hand is not fully resting upon his lap you should remark: "Now your hand is beginning to rise a little." "It is going to rise much more." "See it is continuing to rise."

In case you are wondering what you should do when the subject's arm has risen as far as possible, or as high as desired, you can say the following: "That's fine." "Now let all the normal sensations return to the hand and arm." "Let your arm relax and rest in your lap." "It feels fine, you feel fine."

It is possible that you may encounter a subject whose muscles will lock and who is unable or unwilling to bring his arm down. If this should happen, have him close his eyes and tell him to listen to you carefully. Then proceed to tell him that his arm and hand are becoming relaxed. They are getting heavier and feeling quite normal in every way. If necessary, continue to tell him that his hand and arm are moving back down and he can use them and move them as he normally does. This is an unusually occurrence, put can happen. In any event, never panic. **Remember, what one suggestion can do, other suggestions can undo.**

You should try this experiment on yourself; you will be surprised at the results you get.

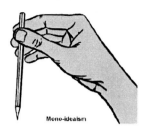
Mono-ideaism

The Pencil Experiment

Figure 5

This is the last experiment we will introduce in this module. Unlike the preceding experiments, this one is not based on ideomotor action. The principle involved here is called "mono-ideaism." Which simply means "one-idea." It is designed to demonstrate how voluntary actions can be inhibited by systematic thinking. When you concentrate on one idea, without interruption, it is virtually impossible to perform the most simple of voluntary actions. The value of this will become apparent when we talk about physical relaxation in later modules. When you can inhibit muscular activity with your thoughts, you can bring on relaxation with your thoughts.

We have called this the pencil experiment, but you can use any similar object, a knife, fork, small stick, etc. Hold the object you intend to use between your thumb and first finger as shown in figure 5. If you decide to drop the object you could do so very easily. All you need to do is open your fingers and it would fall to the ground. Now lets see how easy it is to inhibit the neural processes controlling the fingers holding the object and block the nerve impulses necessary to activate the fingers. We will see if we can make it difficult or impossible for you to drop the object. This inhibitory effect will only last as long as you continue to think as instructed. Your cooperation is vital, make up your mind that you will, for a few seconds, do exactly as instructed.

Hold the object as illustrated in Figure 5. Position your hand so that you can easily observe it and hold it steady for a few minutes. Now, stare at some point on the object, without removing your eyes from it. While you continue to stare at the spot, think to yourself, "I can drop it. I can drop it." Repeat these words over and over with out interruption. During the time you are thinking in this manner you can try to drop the object, but you will find you cannot! It is impossible for you to drop the object if you are thinking the phrase as instructed, over and over without interruption. After experimenting with this a few times you will realize that thinking you can do something does not necessarily mean you can actually do it. In this experiment you have been thinking very intently about dropping an object, but while you are so thinking, you cannot do it.

To open your fingers calls for a decision to be made as to when you want to do it. Making such a decision requires mental activity be instigated in your cerebral cortex. This cannot easily occur when you are exclusively thinking of only one idea. Even if it is the idea of the act you wish to perform.

If you should drop the object, it means one of two things. You are not cooperating, or you have misunderstood the instructions. Reread the instructions and try the experiment again.

MODULE 7 -- WAKING SUGGESTIONS

Backward Postural Sway

Figure 1

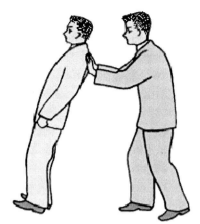

This experiment is only slightly more difficult than the preceding ones. However, you cannot practice this experiment on yourself. If possible you need a subject. If you do not have a helper (subject), you can practice on an imaginary person.

Learning a suggestion also means learning complex coordination of movement and speech. While it is true that mere recitation of suggestions can bring about a desire effect with some subjects, as will be seen later, most situations will require the hypnotist to do a number of other things while giving suggestions. It is very important that such activities are an integral part of the suggestion procedure, and the entire process is as smooth as possible.

Because speed of delivery, intonation, inflection and voice volume are crucial factors, you should practice giving suggestions aloud as much as possible. If you have a tape recorder, it would be a good idea to record your delivery and play it back.

Usually giving suggestions requires that you are standing near the subject, and requires certain motions on your part. Therefore, if you do not have a subject to practice on, you should imagine that you are giving the suggestions to some other person. Role-playing can be extremely useful here. As you continue to practice, you should imagine yourself faced with different situations and change your suggestions accordingly. If possible practice near a full-length mirror. You might use your reflection in the mirror as the subject.

When giving suggestions, your voice and manner should be that of a guide or instructor with no attempt at dominance or control. You should be familiar enough with the entire procedure to retain the over-all concept as you practice. It is not necessary for you to memorize the entire text of the suggestions as given here. Identical wording is not as important as identical meaning.

Although the structure and verbal content of a suggestion is of primary importance, the effectiveness of a suggestion can be greatly improved by a proper use of vocal expression. Quickening of the delivery combined with increasing stress upon critical words in the last half or last third of a suggestion will often increase the response. This is particularly true if there are some indications that the response is beginning to occur. Similarly, changing to an assertive, effective, dynamic expression when the responses are beginning to take place is more effective than continuing in a flat tone of voice. The transition itself has an effect that appears to reinforce the idea that now something is really happening. This not only conveys to the subject that what we have been predicting is now occurring, but the change in our vocal expression indicates to him that we are aware of it, which tends to make it more real to him.

43

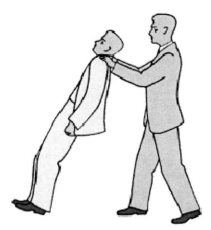

Now, lets assume that you have a person who has volunteered to be a subject. We will also assume that he has little or no knowledge of hypnosis. You might start by saying something like the following to the subject: "I do not know how much knowledge you have about hypnotism, so I would like to tell you a few things about what we are going to do so you will not have any misconceptions about it. First of all, I am not going to put you asleep. I will also tell you if, or when, I intend to hypnotize you. The first thing we are going to do is see how you respond to suggestions. This primarily depends upon how well you are able to cooperate with me. This is not a test of wills. If you have made up your mind to resist, and not to cooperate with me, we might as well quit now. I have absolutely no intention of trying to overcome your will. But if you are willing to cooperate, and do exactly as I ask, we should be able to perform some interesting things. Not only will you find this a very interesting experience, but one that will be beneficial to you in the long run. Before we begin, if you have any questions, I will be glad to answer them." If the subject should have questions, try to briefly answer them. After this, proceed as follows with the experiment.

This experiment is known as "suggested postural sway." In the model suggestions, the words in larger type indicate that they should be said with increased emphasis. This is obtained partly by a rise in voice volume. Smaller type will indicate a decrease in voice volume or emphasis. Emphasis can also be obtained by enunciating each word in a phrase in a staccato fashion. This should be used primarily on text printed in large capitals. We will indicate an increase or decrease in tempo in brackets. The relative length of pauses between words will be indicated by punctuation.

Figure 2

Note: When doing this experiment with a woman wearing high-heeled shoes, ask her to remove her shoes as the heels may snap when she sways backward.

Place yourself about a foot behind the subject. In a normal tone of voice say to him the following:

I would like you to stand before me with your feet together, your arms and hands hanging by your sides... That's right; stand just as you are now. Look straight ahead. Let yourself relax and just listen to me. In a few moments I will ask you to think of falling backwards and shortly after that you will find yourself falling backward. Do not be afraid, I will be behind you and will catch you right away. Do not try to resist. Let me show you how it will feel. [*At this point place yourself no more than a foot from the subject. Place your hands on his shoulders; pull him/her gently but firmly backward (Fig. 2). If necessary, step back a little yourself. Quite often the subject will also step back to prevent himself from falling. If the subject does this, bring him to an upright position keeping your hands on his shoulders and say:*] You stepped back. That is what you must not do. You did it because you were afraid I might let you fall. But you see, I was right here to catch you. Lets try it again. This time let yourself go. Don't be afraid... Alright now, just relax. [*Repeat the above procedure. Usually the subject will let himself fall this time. Even if he does offer some resistance or does step back, continue to say:*] That was better. [*If he did not show any resistance, say:*] Very good. You did very well that time. Now I want you to stand the same way again. Put your heels and toes together and your

44

arms at your sides... Hold your head up straight, [*Place your hand under his chin and tilt his head slightly back*] let your eyelids close and listen closely to what I have to say. [*Proceed in a similar manner if the subject responds correctly the first time. Should he still show some resistance or mistrust, make him aware of this. Reassure him that you will only let him fall a few inches. Repeat this if necessary, and then continue as follows:*] Now I want you to think of yourself as a board, balanced on one end. Think of yourself as falling backward... Imagine you are falling backward, that a force is pulling you backward. In a few moments you will feel a force pulling you backward. Now a force is beginning to pull you backward. You are falling backward... falling backward. Do not resist, let yourself fall. You cannot resist the force. [*Often the subject will show signs of swaying or other signs of responding earlier in the suggestions. If so, shorten the suggestions and proceed to the next part at once. If however, the subject is slow in responding or shows overt resistance, delay the last part and repeat the earlier first part of the suggestions. If the subject should resist, it often helps to interpose this suggestion: "The more you resist, the stronger the force gets, pulling you backward...stronger and stronger."*] You are falling backward, falling, falling, *falling*, FALLING, FALLING...FALL! [*You will usually have to alter this last phase considerable, lengthening it or cutting it short, depending on how the subject is responding, and particularly upon what you anticipate his next response will be.*]

When given the above suggestions, most people will fall backward. A few will waver and sway, but not fall completely. In this case, you should say the following: "You didn't quite fall this time... But you did sway quite a bit. You did feel yourself being pulled back, didn't you? [*Immediately continue with out giving the subject time to answer the question.*] I sensed that you were a little afraid to fall. Let's try it again, but this time let yourself go. Do not be afraid, I am right behind you and will only allow you to fall a few inches. Now put your feet together...."

A few others will step backwards. In this case you should say: "You did not trust me, you stepped back. That is too bad because you would have fallen if you had not stepped back. Let's try it again, but this time try to be relaxed and let yourself fall when you feel yourself being pulled back. Alright now, put your feet together...."

What if your subject did not even sway? Then speak to him in the follow way: "I am afraid you are not cooperating... You must have resisted. Perhaps you are afraid I will let you fall. I assure you I will not. I will be right behind you and only let you fall a few inches. You did feel something, didn't you? [*Again, do not give the subject time to fully answer, but continue to say:*] Now, let's try again, but this time relax. Think only of falling. In your imagination, see yourself falling. Feel yourself falling... don't resist. Just let yourself go. Now think of falling, only falling. Keep thinking of falling..."

In this experiment, as in most of the experiments we have presented, you should keep firing a continuous barrage of suggestions at the subject. **He must not be allowed to think of anything but the desire effect to be produced.** Speak in a normal tone of voice, unless otherwise indicated. Pause, more or less as indicated in the sample suggestions. You want to keep firing suggestions at the subject particularly when he begins to respond. At this point you want to particularly hammer him with suggestions, quicken your delivery and emphasize key words.

In doing this experiment there are three things you should watch for. Sometimes, a subject may tend to fall in the opposite direction. This is very rare, but it does happen, and you must be ready to catch him

45

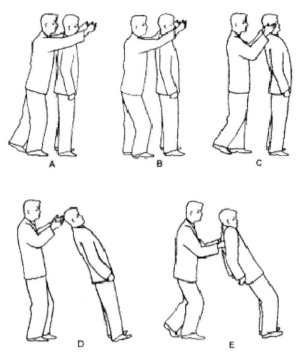

no matter which way he falls. Also, on rare occasions, you may encounter a subject that responds strongly almost immediately. If you are not watching for this you can get caught off balance. The last thing you must watch for are people that have some nervous condition that causes them to lose there balance when they close their eyes. The direction of their fall is unpredictable.

There are many variations of this experiment. For example, in the sample suggestions given above, we asked the subject to close his eyes. Usually closing of the eyes will increase the response, but it is not necessary. You can stand in front of the subject as you explain to him what you expect of him, have him close his eyes or leave them open, and then stand behind him. In the procedure outlined above, we tilted the subject's head slightly back. This is not necessary, but does shift his center of gravity further back, so he is more easily thrown off balance.

Usually you should only try this experiment twice, unless the subject shows definite evidence of responding the second time. Then try it a third time. Of course, if you are doing the experiment for practice, you can try it as often as you like, or until you or your helper get bored or tired. If your subject does not respond the second time, you should try different suggestions. If the subject shows a good response to other suggestions, then return to this one at a later time. As you will learn in a later module, the backward postural sway experiment can be turned into an extraordinarily rapid method of inducing hypnosis.

Some Variations

The following variation of the backward sway experiment is very effective, but is somewhat more difficult to perform.

Figure 3

As before have the subject stand in front of you. Move close to him, almost touching him. Extend your arms outward on both sides of his head as close as possible without touching him. Position your hands level with his eyes, and curve your fingers slightly inward so that the subject can fix his eyes on them (Fig 3A). Extend your hands forward as far a possible and say: "Look at the tips of my fingers. Now, I want you to think of falling backward. In your imagination see yourself falling backward. In a moment I will pull my hands backward; as I do so, you will feel a force pulling you backward. Continue to watch my fingers. As I pull my hands backward [**start to do this very slowly**], you will feel a force pulling you backward. Now the force is beginning to pull you backward. Soon you will fall backward. You are falling backward. A strong force is pulling you backward. You are falling backward. A force

46

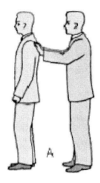 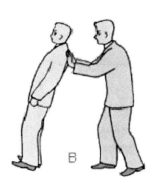

is pulling you... more and more... stronger and stronger. You are falling backward, falling, *falling*, FALLING, FALLING, FALL!." All the time you are speaking, you should be pulling your hands backward. At first, very slowly, then more quickly. This is accomplished by flexing the elbows outward (Fig. 3B). As you do this prepare yourself to step backward as your hands approach the subject's face (Fig. 3C). By this time, if you are successful, the subject should be swaying backward and you will be near the end of the suggestion. As your hands pass swiftly by the side of the subject's face, you should have finished stepping backward (Fig. 3D). At this point, give the emphatic command "FALL!". Then immediately, position your hands to catch the subject (Fig. 3E).

This variation requires considerable coordination between what is said and done. Also timing is very crucial here. However, it is a very effective method that combines a number of effective devices. The fixing of the subject's eyes on the fingers is used to focus his attention. It probably does not produce any degree of hypnosis, as it is not allowed to persist long enough. Indirectly it does aid in the effect of backward motion. The movement itself acts as an additional nonverbal suggestion. Also the subject may reflexively try to avoid the approaching hands by leaning backward or at least tilting his head further back. This would displace his center of gravity in a favorably way. The subject probably does not recognize his avoidance response and confounds it with the expected suggested sway. Therefore, his attitude and suggestibility may also be indirectly positively influenced.

Another, simple variation of this procedure is to stand a foot or so behind the subject, and place the palms of your hands against his shoulder blades as illustrated in Figure 4A.

Figure 4

Your hands should be situated so that your finger tips point toward the top of the subject's shoulders. The remainder of the procedure is much the same as we did before, except that after the introductory instructions you say: "As I pull my hands back from your shoulders you will feel a force pulling you backward." As you do pull your hands back, do it very slowly, maintaining contact with the subject's body until you detect a definite sway (FIG. 4B).

Another variation of the backward sway is to face the subject and ask him to look into your eyes. Then fixate your eyes upon the bridge of his nose. Stand far enough from him to be able to take at least one step forward. Now say to him something like this: "Keep looking into my eyes. Very soon you will feel a force pushing you backward. Think of falling backward... You are going to feel a force pushing you backward. A force is pushing you backward, the force is getting stronger... pushing you backward. You are beginning to feel a force pushing you backward, forcing you back... forcing you to fall. You are going to fall. You are falling backward... etc." If you do not want to have the subject fixate on your eyes, you can have him fixate on your finger. Hold your finger above and slightly in front of your head, so the subject has to look up at it (Fig. 5A). Give suggestions of falling backward as in previous examples. Slowly begin to bring your finger toward the subjects face (Fig5B). In this experiment it

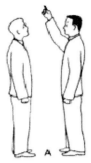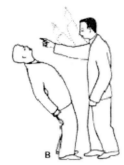

probably would be a good idea to have an assistant available to catch the subject as you may find this difficult to do.

Figure 5

All of the model suggestions we have presented so far have contained a lot of repetition. This is not always necessary. It is possible to get a desired result without a lengthy repetition of suggestions. Sometimes only one single statement is all that is needed. A very effective technique consists of saying to the subject: "I want you to listen carefully to what I am going to say to you. I am going to count from three down to one. At the count of one you will feel an irresistible urge to fall backward. Do not be afraid to fall, I will catch you. Alright now, three...two...ONE! FALL!" The degree of success you have with this technique depends on the degree of suggestibility of the subject. This technique is best used after the subject has shown good responses to a variety of other suggestions.

It is not uncommon for a subject to go into a trance or semitrance during the falling response. When this occurs, the subject usually appears to be unstable on his legs when he is helped to his feet after falling. He may sway and appear "tipsy" or somewhat dazed. If this occurs, unless you want to take advantage of the situation in order to produce a deep trance, snap your fingers near his face and say in a loud voice: "Wake up! You are wide awake, feeling fine." Converse with him a few moments to make sure he is fully awake. ***When giving any kind of suggestion you should always make sure when you are finished that the subject is fully awake and that there are no aftereffects of your suggestions.***

MODULE 8 -- WAKING SUGGESTIONS

HAND CLASPING

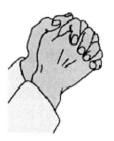

Before you begin these experiments, request that your subjects remove any rings they may be wearing from their fingers. If you do not do this, there is the possibility that they may bruise their fingers.

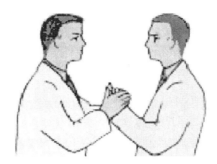

Figure 1

Face your subject and say:

I want you to clasp your hands in this manner... [***Demonstrate to the subject by clasping your hands in front of you, fingers interlocked as shown in Figure 1.***] Now look at my eyes and clasp your hands tightly together. Now I will count from three down to one, at the count of one, let your eyes close and relaxThree...two...one, eye lids closed and relax. [***At this point take hold of his hands and pull them forward, unless they are already extended. Momentarily hold and squeeze his hands together. See Figure 2***]

Figure 2

Make them real tight, *just as tight as you can.* As you continue to tighten your hands you will soon find that your fingers are locking together, your hands are becoming stuck together. Your fingers are locking tighter and tighter, your fingers are sticking together more and more. Your hands are becoming more and more tightly clasped. Your fingers are sticking together. Your hands are sticking together. Your fingers are locked. YOUR HANDS ARE LOCKED TOGETHER; YOU CANNOT TAKE THEM APART. In a moment I will ask you to try to take your hands apart, but *you will not be able to do this.* Your fingers are *absolutely locked* together; your hands are *so complete stuck* together that YOU CANNOT PULL THEM APART. Try. You cannot take them apart. The more you try to take them apart, the more tightly they stick together. Your hands are firmly stuck together...Try hard, you *cannot*, you CAN'T take them apart.

When your subject is trying to meet your challenge, you should give your suggestions in rapid succession. If the subject responds well to the suggestions, you will usually not have to continue giving suggestions. The subject will still not be able to separate his hands.

It is important that you do not allow the subject to feel at any time he could successfully meet your challenge. If you see he is having some success separating his hands or suspect that he will, immediately say: "Now you can separate your hands, everything is as before." Then immediately say to the subject in a positive tone of voice, "You had a little bit of trouble separating your hands, didn't you...They felt kind of struck. Let's try the experiment again." It is very important to say this if the subject did have some difficulty. In no circumstances should you ever appeared dismayed at the results of an experiment. It should always appear that whatever happened was exactly what you expected and wanted.

If the subject should try to separate his hands before you issue your challenge, which may happen, you should point this out to him before trying the experiment again. Emphasize that he is to listen closely to your instructions and carry them out as you give them and not anticipate your instructions. Anticipatory reactions are often a sign of resistance or noncooperation on the part of a subject. If you have reason to believe that the subject was not cooperating, it should be pointed out. Explain to him that the success of the suggestions depend upon his cooperation. Sometimes you will find that subjects resist by weakly clasping their hands. This is one reason for holding their hands at the beginning of the experiment. This allows you to determine how tightly they are clasping their hands. If a subject fails to follow your instructions, you may have to be more assertive. You might say: "Come on, you can do better than that! Clasp your hands real tight, *tight*, JUST AS TIGHT AS YOU CAN!" At the same time strongly squeeze his hands together to emphasize your instructions. Even if he should then tighten his clasp, it is no guarantee he will maintain a tight grasp. Some noncooperative subjects will proceed to relax their hands before or at the time of the challenge. In this case you should again point out his obvious resistance to the suggestions. You will find that some subjects, despite their desire to cooperate, tend to respond in a passive way giving the appearance of noncooperation. The following variation of the handclasp experiment seems to work very well with them.

Tell your subject the following:I want you to clasp your hands like this...Look at my eyes and clasp your hands tightly together... Make them real tight, AS TIGHT AS YOU CAN! Think of your hands as tightly clasped together, feel your fingers pressing down upon the backs of your hands, feel your hands becoming more and more tightly clenched together. [*Continue holding the subject's hands. If they are not tightly clasped, continue to say:* "as you do so and continue to listen to what I say you will find that your fingers tend to close...to press against the backs of your hands, that your hands are being pressed tightly together. You are unable to help yourself." Else go on with what follows while gently letting go of the subjects hands.] Your hands are being tightly stuck together; your fingers are pressing your hands tightly together. Now your fingers and hands are becoming *stiff, rigid...more and more stiff. Your hands are stuck tightly together. So tightly that you cannot take them apart.* THEY ARE STUCK TOGETHER! YOU CANNOT SEPARATE THEM! Try! YOU CANNOT! YOU CAN'T SEPARATE THEM! THE MORE YOU TRY THE TIGHTER THEY ARE STUCK TOGETHER!

There are several things about the above procedures that should be pointed out. The subject's arms should be well extended out when doing the handclasp experiment. There is a degree of leverage in our favor when the arms are extended. The muscles involved are those used to rotate the arm about the shoulder. The further the arms are extended, the less leverage these muscles have against any force preventing the hands moving laterally outward (pulling apart). There is another mechanical advantage to this experiment. While the hands are tightly clasp, the joints of the fingers, due to their shape, tend to lock the hands together and prevent the fingers from sliding apart. For this reason you should make sure that the base of the fingers are against one another.

After reading the above paragraph you may get the impression that this experiment is based on a mechanical illusion and deception. This is not true. If a subject is not suggestible, he will simply relax his hands before or shortly after trying to pull them apart. This is not the situation if he is responding to suggestions. The subject will tighten his hands to a considerable degree as you give suggestions. In fact with a very suggestible subject you can start with his hands clasped loosely and his hands fairly close to his body.

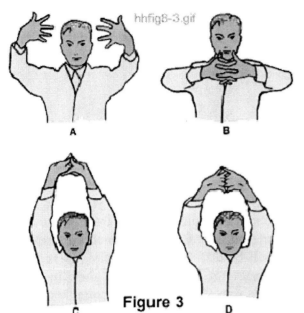

Figure 3

Many subjects will respond very strongly to hand clasping suggestions. In fact they may respond so strongly that you can challenge then repeatedly to separate their hands. They will make all kind of contortions trying to get their hands apart all to no avail. They will not be able to get their hand apart *until you tell you them they can.* In this case you can end the response by snapping your fingers and saying: "Alright now, relax. You can take your hands apart now. They are not stuck anymore." Even after this some subject may still have some difficulty separating their hands. If this happens, take hold of their wrists and pull their hands apart saying again: "Your hands are relaxed now,...you can easily separate your hands." Incidentally, such individuals will nearly always make very good subjects for hypnotic experiments. Almost invariably, most people that respond well to hand clasping suggestions can be hypnotized fairly deeply and with little difficulty.

Chinese Handclasp

The following is a variation of the hand clasping experiment. Have your subject extend his hands and arms in front of him, palms facing one another. Now tell him to bend his hands so the palms face him and the tips of the fingers are opposite each other (Fig. 3A). Next have him spread his fingers apart and bring his hands together so the fingers interlock and touch at the base (palms still apart). See Figure 3B. Now tell him to rotate his hands so he sees the backs of his hands (Fig.3C). Finally, have him elevate his hands above his head, palms outward and his arms outstretched as much as possible (Fig. 3D).

Demonstrate the procedure as you as you tell him what to do. Then have him go through the procedure, step by step. Then say to him:

Please look into my eyes and listen carefully to what I tell you. Keep your hands above your head, arms extended and fingers interlocked. Think of your arms stiffening and your fingers becoming tight. As I speak your fingers and hands are becoming tight. Your arms are becoming stiff...Think of nothing else...The muscles of your arms and hands are becoming more and more tight, stiff. Your hands are getting tighter and tighter, your arms are becoming stiffer and stiffer. I am going to count from one down to three; at the count of three you will not be able to unlock your hands and fingers. One...Your hands are getting tight, very tight, so tight you cannot separate them. Two...Your hands and arms are getting stiff, stiffer, so stiff you can't move them. THREE...*your hands are stuck. Your fingers are locked together.* YOU CANNOT TAKE YOUR HANDS APART, the more you try the tighter they become stuck. Try...You CANNOT...The more you try the tighter they stick together.

51

Some hypnotists prefer to give the above suggestions with the subjects eyes closed. Both methods seem equally effective. The important thing in this experiment is that nothing distracts the subject's attention from the suggestions.

Wolberg's Method

Another variation has been described by Wolberg. It differs from the other methods in that he makes use of the subject's imagination. He usually has the subject sit down and clasp his hands. He then says:

I want you to close your eyes for a moment and visualize a vise, a heavy metal vise whose jaws clamp together with a screw. Imagine that your hands are like the jaws of the vise, and as you press them together tighter, they are just like the jaws of the vise tightening. I am going to count from one to five. As I count your hands will press together tighter, and tighter, and tighter. When I reach the count of five, your hands will be pressed together so firmly that it will be difficult or impossible to separate them. One, tight; two, tighter and tighter and tighter; three, very tight, your hands are glued together; four, your hands are clamped tight, tight; five, so tight that even though you try to separate them, they remain clasped together, until I give you the command to open them -- Now open them slowly.

Eye Catalepsy

The term "catalepsy" actually refers to a state of muscular rigidity in which a person's body retains any position it may be given. However, it is used rather indiscriminately by hypnotists to cover a number of situations. It's common to use it to refer to any muscular condition in which a subject is unable to voluntarily move any part of his body or his entire body. In any event, we will use it to describe "eye catalepsy" as well as the other "catalepsies" regardless of their nature since it is a well-established terminology in hypnotic literature. Stand next to your subject and say:

Please close your eyes and relax. Don't be afraid, I am not going to hypnotize you yet. [*As soon as he complies, place your finger on the top of his forehead.*] Keep your eyes closed tight and turn your eyes upward as though you were looking through the top of your forehead at the tip of my finger. Keep your eyes tightly closed and keep looking upward. As you do so, you will find that your eyelids are becoming heavy and closing more tightly. They are closing more and more tightly and becoming very heavy, very heavy. They are sticking closed. Shortly I will tell you to try to open your eyes, but you will find this very difficult to do, very hard, because your eyelids are being stuck just as if they were glued shut. They feel very heavy, like lead. They are stiff. They are stuck. They are sticking tighter and tighter. They are heavy as lead. Your eyelids are sticking closed, as if glued closed. They are stuck closed. Your eyes are sticking closed. They are stuck closed, YOU CANNOT OPEN YOUR EYES!...*the more you try the more stuck they become.*

Sometimes when a person looks upward he may not be able to completely close his eyes. Therefore, you may find that some subjects show an appreciable slit, or after they begin to respond to your suggestions they tend to lift their eyelids a little. Do not be concerned about this. Just repeat your request that they keep their eyes closed and keep looking upward. By watch the rolling of his eyes under the eyelids, you can usually tell how well the subject is looking upward. Some subjects may complain that it hurts their eyes or that they cannot do both, look up and close their eyes tightly. In such cases ask them to look up the best that they can without discomfort, but with their eyes closed.

A person that is somewhat suggestible will experience considerable difficulty opening his eyes. If he does succeed, but shows some difficulty, you should point it out to him. As with the hand clasping experiments, if it looks like the subject is going to overcome the suggestion, quickly say: "Alright, stop trying, you can open your eyes."

Frequently, when asked to close their eyes, subjects assume this is a preliminary step to the induction of hypnosis. If they are not ready for this, they may build up resistance because of anxiety. For this reason the subject should be told at the beginning that he is not going to be hypnotized. Note in the above example that we said: "I am not going to hypnotize you *yet*..." This is not the same a saying to him: "I am not going to hypnotize you." or "I will not hypnotize you with out telling you first." The first statement will reassure the subject, but says nothing about the near future. If you should hypnotize the subject later, he will be less likely to feel he has been tricked, and that you can't be trusted. Also, if you tell the subject: "I am not going to hypnotize you." it could act as a counter-suggestion to later suggestions leading to an induction of hypnosis. Later you will see that eye catalepsy can be made a part of a trance induction technique.

Arm Catalepsy

Have your subject hold his arm horizontally straight out at his side, form a fist and look into your eyes. Hold his fist, squeeze it lightly, and pull his arm outward. While you are doing this, with your other arm grasp his forearm and speak to him as follows: "Think of your arm as stiff and rigid, stiff like a steel bar. Your arm is becoming stiff, *stiffer* and *stiffer*. It is becoming stiff like a bar of steel, ridge as a piece of iron. In a moment it will be so *stiff* and *rigid* that you will be unable to bend it or move it. Your arm is now *stiff* and *rigid...like a rod of steel. You can't bend your arm, you cannot move it.* TRY. YOU CAN'T!...etc."

Making the Hands Heavy or Stuck

Have your subject sit comfortably with his hand resting in his lap. Fixate your gaze on the bridge of his nose and say to him: "Look at my eyes and follow my instructions carefully. Soon you will find that your [right or left] hand is becoming heavy. It will get heavier and heavier, so heavy that you will not be able to lift it when I ask you to try. For now just listen to my voice. Your hand is beginning to feel heavy. A feeling of heaviness is flowing into your hand and back into your arm. Your arm and hand are becoming very heavy...heavier and heavier. Your hand feels very heavy...your arm feels very heavy. They are now very heavy...v-e-r-y h-e-a-v-y, *just like lead.* They are so h-e-a-v-y that you cannot lift your hand. *Your hand feels as though it were stuck to your lap. You cannot lift it!* YOU CANNOT! Try! YOU CAN'T! The more you try, the heavier you hand becomes."

Making the Subject Unable to Drop an Object

If you succeeded in getting a strong response in the hand clasping experiment, you will nearly always succeed with this experiment. Especially, if you also got a good response to the eye catalepsy or arm rigidity experiment. Give the subject some object (i.e. a spool of thread) to hold in one hand in such a manner that if he opens his hand the object will fall to the floor. Have him fix his gaze on your eyes and firmly say to him: "Hold the spool tightly. I am going to count from three down to one; at the count of one you will find it impossible to let go of the spool. You will not be able to drop it. Your hands and fingers are going to be stuck to the spool...Three...your hand is sticking to the spool; your fingers are becoming stuck to the spool. Your hand and fingers are now stuck to the spool. They are sticking tighter and tighter, so tight you cannot open your hand no matter how hard you try. Two...Your hand and fingers are now stuck fast to the spool. They are sticking tight, so tight you can't open your hand. ONE!...*Your hand is struck to the spool, your fingers are stuck to it!* YOU CANNOT DROP IT! Try! YOU CAN'T. YOU CAN'T OPEN YOUR HAND."

Forcing the Release of an Object

Have the subject hold the spool as described above and instruct him to hold it tightly. Fixate him and give suggestions that he will not be able to hold on to the spool. The more he tries to hold on to the spool the less able he is to do so. Tell him that his hand is opening, that the spool is repelling his fingers, forcing them open, that he cannot hold on to the spool, etc.

The Arm Twirl Experiment
Figure 4

Tell the subject to hold his arms and hands as illustrated in Figure 4. Then tell him to twirl them away from himself and around each other slowly like he would do if he were twiddling his thumbs. (Note: the thumbs could be used in this experiment instead of the arms.) Then suggest to the subject that when he tries to stop twirling his arms he will not be able to do so. Suggest that his arms are twirling faster and faster, etc.

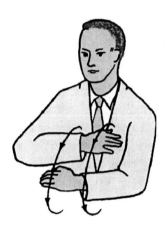

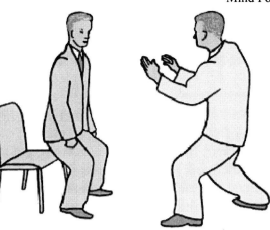

Forcing a Subject to Sit

Have the subject stand in front of a chair in a way that he could easily sit in it. Have him fixate on your eyes and say to him: "Think of sitting down. I will count from three down to one, at the count of one you will find your legs feeling very weak, your knees will fold, you will feel so heavy that you will have to sit down...Three...two...one! You are becoming heavier and heavier...heavier...Your knees are folding...your legs are getting weak...Your knees are folding, folding...Your body is heavy...Your body is going down, down...You are sitting down...sitting down...etc.

Figure 5

As soon as you see any response from the subject, you should partially bend your knees and lower your body slowly downward. Also it is very effective to hold your hands up, palms facing the subject and at the right moment slowly lower them in a suggestive manner. The two techniques can be combined to enhance each other. See Figure 5. If the subject is not responding it is helpful to use these techniques at the time you tell the subject his body is going down.

Causing the Subject to Hallucinate Heat

Responses to motor suggestions are by far the easiest to achieve in the waking state. Sensory hallucinations and distortions can also be produced but are more difficult to produce. Probably the easiest sensory effect to produce is the illusion of heat. For this you need a subject that has responded well to the experiment given above. Ask your subject to hold his hand out horizontally, palm up. Place a small coin in his palm. Have him look at the coin and say: "Shortly this coin is going to begin to get warm. You will feel it get warm...warmer...warmed and warmer, then hot. [*If your subject is very suggestible, this will be sufficient to produce the sensation of heat. The subject will drop the coin and report that it got very hot. If this does not occur, then continue.*] Now the coin is getting warmer...warmer...warmer...You can feel it getting warmer, don't you? *It is now very warm,...in fact it is getting hot...very hot...hotter...*HOTTER...RED HOT!"

Producing Anesthesia

The hallucination of heat as in the above experiment is called a *positive* hallucination. The reverse of this is called a negative hallucination. One of the easiest negative hallucinations to produce is suggested anesthesia for pain. Have your subject sit comfortably in a chair, his hand on his lap. Have him fixate on his hand and tell him that in a moment his hand will become numb and he will be unable to feel any pain. Then continue with:

Now let your eyelids close and listen carefully to my voice. Shortly all feeling will be gone from your hand. You will not be able to feel anything with your hand. Think of your hand as getting numb...as though it were going to sleep. As you keep this thought in mind, you will find your hand is becoming numb. With every sound of my voice, your hand is becoming more and more numb...You can feel less and less, your hand is losing all feeling. Very soon you will be unable to feel any pain in your hand. You will feel absolutely no pain. I will count from three down to one; at the count of one your hand will be totally insensible to pain. You will be unable to feel pain...Three...your hand is becoming insensitive to pain...you are losing all feeling. It is getting very numb, more numb. You can feel less and less with your hand and you are losing awareness of it. Soon you will be unable to feel anything with your hand. Two...*Your hand is becoming number.* There is very little feeling in it. It feels like it was asleep. *It is impossible to feel any pain in it, it is completely numb.* One...*Your hand is completely without feeling.* YOU CANNOT FEEL ANY PAIN...NO MATTER WHAT I DO. YOU CAN'T FEEL ANY PAIN.

The standard test for anesthesia is to lift a flap of skin on the back of the subject's hand and pierce it with a sterile pin or needle. When using waking suggestions it is best to keep suggesting to the subject that he feels no pain as the needle passes through the skin. It is also a good idea to suggest that there will be no after-pain after the needle is removed.

Many other kinds of hallucinations can be induced in the waking state. However, the best results are obtained with hypnotized subjects. Therefore, we will leave further discussions for inducing hallucinations until later. In general, the techniques for inducing hallucinations in the waking state and in hypnosis are essential the same. Usually in the waking state it is necessary to give longer and more elaborate suggestions than in hypnosis. You can often say to a hypnotized individual: "At the snap of my finger you will feel very warm -- very hot," and get a positive response. With waking suggestions you have to go more slowly. Waking individuals, as a rule, tend to give weaker responses to suggestions (there are exceptions). The responses to waking suggestions also tend to be more temporary than those elicited under hypnosis. This will conclude our discussions on waking suggestions. In the next module (module 9) we will discuss suggestions in general and in module 10 we will discuss hypnosis and hypnotic suggestions.

MODULE 9 -- SUGGESTION IN GENERAL

Integrating and Combining Suggestions

Suggestions can be given individually, independently of one another, but it is often advantageous to give several suggestions sequentially as a continuous unit. It not only makes a more effective demonstration, but also often has a facilitative effect on some of the suggestions in the unit.

Training the Subject

Each individual has a maximal potentiality for response to suggestions. Part of this is innate, and part is acquired. Very few individuals initially manifest their maximal potential suggestibility. This is partly due to interfering factors such as attitudes, beliefs and anxiety. The induction of hypnosis by the Standard method requires that a certain degree of suggestibility is present at the beginning. In a similar way, the success of each waking suggestion calls for a minimal amount of suggestibility. In both cases it may be necessary to increase the subject's initial suggestibility in order to achieve a desire effect. This preliminary step is usually referred to in hypnotic literature as "training" the subject. Homoaction and heteroaction are the two basic processes that are used for this purpose. Based on their properties the following procedural rules have been established: When you begin working with a subject, especially the first time, you should give him a number of different suggestions in rapid succession. Each should contain many repetitions of the suggested idea. If a response is weak or absent, it should be given at least once again. Always proceed from the simpler to the more complex (easier to the more difficult) suggestion. Always give motor suggestions first and sensory suggestions later. Your objective should always be for a strong, well-defined and complete response to your suggestions. For this reason it is important that you do not tax the subject's suggestibility. If you start with a suggestion that calls for greater suggestibility than the subject has, you will get neither homoaction nor heteroaction. If he responds weakly or incompletely, the heteroaction if not the homoaction will suffer. This is true even if the inadequate response occurs someplace in a sequence of successful suggestions. In fact, because of the summarized nature of heteroaction, failure to respond to a suggestion will tend to extinguish or decrease the heteroaction gained at this point.

There are other benefits from following the above rules. A successful suggestion always tends to increase the hypnotist's prestige and to create in the subject a more positive attitude toward his ability to affect the subject. A rapid succession of suggestions tends to keep the subject's attention focused upon the hypnotist.

It is possible to raise a subject's suggestibility, without taxing his responsiveness, by giving him a series of suggestions of equal difficulty or complexity. One problem with this approach is you will very quickly run out of suggestions. Also, because the goal is to increase his suggestibility, it is desirable to have an idea just what his suggestibility is at any given time. Both problems can be solved by using a set of suggestions graded in the degree of suggestibility needed to elicit a satisfactory response. Start with the suggestion having the lowest requirement and progress to the one with the highest requirement. At any time the subject should give a weak, unsatisfactory, or no response, to a suggestion, take this as an indication that his suggestibility has not or has barely reached the level needed for that suggestion. Should the response be a weak one, you can then repeat the previous suggestions or introduce new ones of similar difficulty. Eventually retest the subject with the failed suggestion.

The suggestions given in previous modules, Chevreul's pendulum, backward postural sway, hand levitation, hand clasping, and eye catalepsy constitute a set of graded suggestions in the order low to high suggestibility. The recommended procedure is to start with the Chevreul pendulum and rapidly work up through the remaining suggestions given above. Another reason for doing this is to get an idea how susceptible an individual is to hypnosis. With a little experience you will find you can skip certain suggestions when you have a subject who is obviously very suggestible. However, as a rule, unless there is evidence that a subject is very suggestible, go rapidly through the postural sway, hand clasping, and eye catalepsy suggestions, especially if you intend to induce hypnosis.

Increased Suggestibility Via Voluntary Action

There is a lot of evidence that suggests *voluntarily* executing a given action facilitates its subsequent re-execution. This means your suggestion is likely to be more effective if shortly before giving it, you have been able to get the subject to voluntarily perform the suggested act. This is one of the factors involved in the hand clasping experiment. Remember, we had the subject voluntarily stiffen his hands. Many hypnotists believe that getting the subject to voluntarily do a number of simple things can facilitate not only repeated responses, but also future suggestions. A simple way to do this is to move the subject about under the guise of procedure. You can ask him to stand here...or better here...no, turn like this, etc. As soon as you are through with an experiment, you can have the subject sit down. Then shortly afterward, have him stand up for another experiment. If you are going to hypnotize him, have him move to another chair. If he crosses his legs after sitting down, you can ask him to uncross them. All of this must appear as natural and not be overdone.

The efficient use of voluntary responses can be nicely demonstrated by describing a procedure for hand clasping used by the late stage hypnotist Konradi Leitner. He used the Chinese hand clasping experiment as a group or mass suggestion. His objective was to *insensibly transform* voluntary responses into responses to waking suggestions and these into responses in a light to medium state of hypnosis.

Leitner would start by making brief introductory remarks that were designed to create a receptive attitude and establishing rapport with the audience. The audience was then asked to stand up. Sufficient time was allowed for everyone to stand. At the same time with the instructions to stand up, he would straighten himself, suggesting nonverbally that the audience should do the same. The audience was then instructed to remove everything from their hands and to relax. Again sufficient time was allowed for the audience to remove rings, handbags, purses, cigarettes, etc., from their hands. Leitner then instructed the audience to inhale deeply and to hold their breath for ten seconds. He would then say at the count of ten "Exhale slowly." This was repeated three times. Leitner also inhaled, held his breath in unison with the audience. In order to accentuate this procedure he would also hold his hands and arms outstretched in front of his chest, horizontal and parallel to each other, fingers spread with palms down. With each inhalation he would raise both arms slightly above the level of his forehead. They were held in this position for the duration of the ten-second pause. They were then lowered to the horizontal position in unison with the exhalation. This procedure served two purposes: it introduced a nonverbal suggestion, by example, of the voluntary act of breathing, helped to show the audience what was desired of them. The arm motion served as a suggestion and as a means of emphasizing and controlling the action asked for.

At the end of the third command to exhale, he would give the instructions for the hand clasping experiment (see module 8). He would slowly demonstrate each step. He added an additional step to the procedure that we did not use in module 8. When the audience had their arms extended with their fingers spread (Module .8, Fig. 3A) he would instruct them to breathe again deeply and then to exhale slowly. In the next step he had them again breathe deeply, but this time he would add, "as you inhale, raise your arms." At the same time he raised his. Then as soon as the audience complied, he would instruct them to lower their arms slowly and exhale.

The above procedure was repeated three times. The audience was next instructed to interlock their fingers and turn their palms outward. This was demonstrated to the audience slowly step by step. This not only makes it very clear to the audience exactly what they are expected to do, but has them perform a series of voluntary responses which serves as a foundation upon which to build up the audience's suggestibility. When properly done, it allows the hypnotist to pass insensibly from the elicitation of voluntary acts to suggestion proper.

With their fingers interlocked and their hands turned outward, the audience was instructed to take another deep breath, hold it for ten seconds, then exhale. Then they were asked, while keeping their hands interlocked, to synchronize their breathing with movements of their arms from the horizontal to above their heads. After the audience preformed this exercise a few times he would tell them in a few moments they would be asked to close their eyes. He would then in quick succession command them sharply to raise their arms overhead, breath deeply, and to close their eyes. He would then say: "Your eyes are closed. Now breath deeply..in unison. Keep your hands over your head...Your hands and fingers are interlocked...Breathe deeply, in harmony...Now your hands are beginning to become tight...I shall begin to count to three. As I count your hands will get tighter and tighter and when I reach the count of three you will not be able to unlock your hands and fingers...Breathe in unison...I shall now begin to count...One...Your hands begin to feel tight...Two...Your arms and your hands are becoming stiff...Three...You cannot take your hands apart. Try. You cannot unlock your hands."

Essentially this was Leitner's way of demonstrating the hand clasping exercise. He very skillfully blended actual suggestions with other instructions. The entire procedure was designed to secure the maximum attention of the audience and to keep it focused upon the suggestions and instructions. He kept the audience executing voluntary actions (or at least what were initially voluntary actions) throughout the entire procedure. This is an excellent technique especially well suited for mass hypnosis. He usually passed from the hand clasping suggestions to the induction of hypnosis proper.

Note that Leitner extensively used deep rhythmic breathing as part of his procedure. Many hypnotists feel that deep breathing directly helps in inducing and deepening the trance state. Some experimental evidence does seem to indicate that deep breathing (hyperventilation) does have a positive affect upon a subject's suggestibility, but as a whole the available evidence is poor.

The Counting Technique

There are occasions when what appears to be a potentially good subject responds poorly. This is often the case with passive subjects (see below). In these cases the so-called "counting technique" can be very effective. We have used it in several of our previous experiments; it can be used in any situation. With very suggestible subjects it can be very effective. You only need to say: "At the count of three you will do so and so...One...Two...Three." and the suggestion takes effect. With subjects that have failed to give a response, or that have given a weak response, better results can often be obtained by stating very positively: "Now I am going to count to three and at the count of three, such and such will happen. You will not be able to prevent it. In fact if you did try, you would find it happens more strongly. Alright now, One...Two...THREE!" In some situations you may feel that a longer count is necessary. You can also add suggestions at the end of each count. Varying situations call for varying techniques.

Passive Subjects

Quite often you will encounter subjects that appear to be potentially excellent subjects, but who do poorly when given many of the suggestions. They respond well to the falling back experiment and are easily hypnotized, but in other respects they are rather unresponsive. Such individuals are known as *passive* subjects. They often show a disinclination to exert any muscular effort when asked to do so. When challenged, they probably will do nothing at all. For demonstrations or experimental work, it is best not to use them. However, for therapeutic purposes, these individuals can be extremely suggestible and the use of hypnosis can be very effective. How should these subjects be handled? -- I don't know. The use of a more positive, commanding, authoritarian approach will sometimes overcome their passivity to some degree. The counting technique above can be very effective. The subject may have various personal reasons for behaving the way he does which can be uncovered by questioning him. The causes can then be eliminated or circumvented. The point I wish to make is that unresponsiveness or what appears to be unresponsiveness on the part of a subject is not always an indication of low suggestibility.

Sometimes subjects react to suggestions in a way that is very perplexing for the hypnotist. One reaction that sometimes occurs with waking suggestions is that the subject smiles, often broadly, when you give your suggestions. This usually occurs when a subject finds himself responding, to his great surprise, to your suggestions. The smiling is nothing more than an expression of his surprise. Very seldom does a subject smile because the situation appears funny to him. In such an event, it is best to ignore the reaction and to continue with the suggestions as if nothing had occurred. There may be exceptions where you feel you must interrupt the proceedings. In such a case you should start over rather than continue from where you quit. If possible try to integrate the subject's actions into the procedures, else ignore them. It is always a good idea to ask the subject at the end of the experiment, why he behaved as he did (i.e., why he smiled).

Nonverbal Suggestions

Nonverbal suggestions are an important complement in giving suggestions. They vary considerably and can be anything from a facial expression, a stance, a tone of voice, to a motion of the entire body.

Although the structure and verbal content of a suggestion is of prime importance, the effectiveness of a suggestion can be greatly enhanced by a proper use of vocal expression. If there is some indication that a response to a suggestion is beginning to take place, changing to an assertive, effective, dynamic expression will increase the response. We not only tell the subject that what we have been predicting is now occurring, but the change in our vocal expression indicates to him our awareness of it, possibly making it more real to him.

Another factor that should be taken into consideration are the vocal expressions of the hypnotist that reflect his feelings, attitudes and emotions. It is important that suggestions be given in a tone of voice that projects conviction, self-assurance and confidence. Within limits, a suggestion will be effective in proportion to the degree to which the hypnotist believes in its effectiveness and the reality of the

60

phenomena it elicited. For example, if the hypnotist wants to suggest disgust he will be more effective if he can make his tone of voice express this, along with his facial expression, posture, etc. If the hypnotist says to the subject: "You feel disgusted," and at the same time he expresses disgust in his tone of voice and shows it in his facial expression, we have three different stimuli, each of which have the power to evoke the same response in the subject. They are all working at the same time and mutually reinforcing each other.

Continuity and Discontinuity of Ideas in Suggestions

Frequently when giving suggestions we not only present the idea of the desired effect to the subject, but to precede or accompany it with one or more subsidiary ideas that suggest the effect indirectly. One of the most common ways to do this is by the use of metaphors. For example, when suggesting to a subject whose eyes are closed that he cannot open them, one could assert that his eyelids are heavy, heavy as lead, and that when he tries to open them he will find it impossible to do so because it is as if his eyes were glued tightly shut. Also, when suggesting to a subject that he is falling backward, we often tell him that he is going to fall, but this is so because some strong force is pulling him backward. There are some advantages to doing this. Because the subsidiary ideas indirectly suggest the same end result as the principal idea, it is assumed that there will be some sort of synergetic action. Also, it is possible that the subject might misinterpret what effect is expected and by stating it a variety of ways may lessen the chance of a misunderstanding. Sometimes a subject may be incapable of conceptualizing or visualizing a certain effect when it is stated in one way, but if worded in a different way he has no problem with it. Another advantage to proceeding in this way is that it gives the subject the opportunity to participate more actively in the production of the suggested effect by selecting which idea to act upon.

On the other hand, some hypnotists feel this technique is harmful because it introduces discontinuities in the subject's thoughts. If monoideaism or sustained attention is basic to the production of suggested phenomena, this is a reasonable position to take. To first call the subject's attention to the concept that his eyes are too heavy to open and then to the idea that they are glued closed does appear at first glance to be incompatible with the above conditions. In actual practice you will find that some subjects respond best to suggestions when you adhere to strict continuity of ideas, while others seem to benefit from the introduction of subsidiary ideas. It would be nice to have some idea how individual subject might react to discontinuities of ideas. It has been my experience that people who are literal-minded, that have critical analytical minds, that place a high value on words, that are trained or prone to use a highly precise language are the one that are most frequently unable to tolerate discontinuity or will only tolerate a small amount of it. These people often seem to perceive the subsidiary ideas as being incompatible with one another as well as the central idea of the suggestion, even though no logical or linguistic incompatibility really exists. Their tendency to literalness with regard to the wording of a suggestion often shows up in a different way that is worth calling attention to. For most people it is unimportant when giving a suggestion of eye closure whether you say, "Your eyelids are heavy," or "Yours eyes are heavy." With these subjects this becomes very important. Typically they will tell you that when you tell them their eyes were heavy they found it impossible to conceive of their *eyeballs* being heavy. Not all individuals who perceive incompatibilities between ideas in a suggestion will react this way. Some just ignore all but the idea that appeals to them and allow it to have its effects upon them. My experience has been that the use of subsidiary ideas is most likely to cause difficulties for subjects that are professional scientists.

MODULE 10 -- INDUCTION OF HYPNOSIS

INDUCTION OF HYPNOSIS

The induction of hypnosis consists of three phases:

Preparation
Induction proper
Deepening the trance

The three phases are not separate and distinct; in fact there is considerable overlapping. The first phase (preparation) consists of the elimination of unfavorable factors and the activation of as many favorable ones as possible. The second (induction) consists of inducing a change in the subject that is characterized by passing from the waking state into the hypnotic state. The last (Deepening) consists of maximizing this change.

Because the preparatory and deepening phases are virtually the same regardless of the method used to induce hypnosis, we will only describe them once with the first induction method. After this we will only describe various methods used in the second phase, the reader is expected to remember what has been said concerning the other phases.

A Simple Induction

Preparatory Phase

If you have had access to a number of subjects while performing previous experiments, pick a subject that gave strong responses to your waking suggestions, especially to the postural sway, hand clasping, and eye catalepsy suggestions. Begin with the subject standing near you with a chair near by that is easily accessible to the subject. Tell him that very soon you are going to hypnotize him. Say this in a positive tone of voice with conviction. Never, use expressions such as "I am going to *try*" or "I will now *attempt*" since this implies doubt concerning your ability to induce a trance. At this point a subject may show signs of nervousness or uneasiness. If so, explain to him there is nothing to fear, that he will find this a very pleasant and interesting experience. One that will benefit him greatly. If he still seems disturbed, ask him what is bothering him. Once you know what his concerns are, talk reassuringly to him about them. Some subjects worry about losing consciousness when being hypnotized. Assure them that they will not be unconscious when hypnotized, and will be aware of everything that goes on. As will be seen later, some subjects, consciously or unconsciously, set certain conditions for entering the trance state. In such instances, the conditions must be incorporated into the induction procedure.

It is a good idea to instruct the subject to remain as passive as possible. Tell him to listen to what you say, but not to try to help or resist in any way. Tell him not to try to think about or analyze what he is

62

told will happen or is happening, but just let it happen. Tell him to allow any urge he feels to develop. Tell the subject, "Don't try to do anything or not to do anything -- just let yourself go."

Often it is advantageous to repeat these last instructions as the induction proceeds, particularly if there is evidence that he is resisting or in some way interfering with the induction. A frequent source of difficulty occurs when the subject begins to actively think about and analyze his experiences. Sometimes this occurs when the hypnotist gives instructions or uses words that are not clearly defined for the subject. For example, telling him to make his mind "blank" often leaves the subject uncertain as to how to do this.

As a result he may not know exactly what you want. He may question you as to what you mean by this. You should then explain to him what is desired in words he can understand. Even such a simple thing as relaxing can cause trouble because the subject may not know how to relax. In trying to relax he may tense his muscles.

The main objective of the preparatory phase is to facilitate the induction proper of hypnosis. Because the first technique presented is typical of the Standard method, suggestions play an important part from the beginning. The more suggestible our subject is the more successful we will be in hypnotizing him. Therefore, we want to raise his degree of suggestibility by any mean we can. One-way to accomplish this is to give the subject a set of graded (easy to more difficult) suggestions.

It is essential to only give the subject suggestions that he will respond well to. This is one reason for using a graded series. By starting with the easiest suggestion first, we stand a better chance of getting a good response. Also, if the subject responds, then the chances of his responding to the next harder suggestion may be improved because some heteroaction has occurred. In this way we can gradually build up the subject's suggestibility. Another reason for using a graded series is that it gives you some idea of how suggestible the subject is at any stage of the procedure. Another thing we can do is get the subject to voluntarily do various things. Many hypnotists do this in the preparatory stage.

There is no well-defined boundary between waking and hypnotic suggestibility. Essentially the same processes that are responsible for the development of hypnotic hypersuggestibility can and do become active when a series of waking suggestions are given. For this reason, the preparatory phase tends to blend with the induction proper and it is not uncommon to find that a subject is "partially" hypnotized at the end of the preparatory phrase.

Hypnosis developing before the induction proper is started may cause the novice some concern. Subjects who become hypnotized at this early stage usually do not close their eyes. This occurs despite the fact that eye closure is suggested in the Standard method. Eye closure is not a requirement for hypnosis nor is it a symptom of hypnosis. It is well known that a subject can have his eyes open without affecting the trance when the hypnosis is deep enough. Actually, eye closure only takes place because it is directly or indirectly suggested. Subjects can be easily hypnotized with their eyes remaining open. Reports of Braid, Charcot and many others, indicate that a fixed stare with eyes wide open was originally more a characteristic of hypnosis than closed eyes. However, theoretically eye closure can be useful in light to medium hypnosis because it eliminates distracting stimuli in a purely mechanical way. It is also a relatively easy response to suggestion and is therefore a contributor to the generalization of suggestibility.

Sometimes, for no obvious reason, a subject will unexpectedly open his eyes during hypnosis. This can occur with deeply hypnotized subject, even though instructions have been given to the contrary. Unless the trance was a relatively light one, the subject is probably *still hypnotized*. We emphasize this because many novices interpret this as a failure, when it is not. A simple command to close his eyes or to sleep is usually all that is needed to restore the status quo. It is also a good idea to follow this up with a few suggestions aimed at deepening the trance. In some case when the subject seems definitely awake it is possible to bring back the trance state to its former depth if suggestions are given quickly.

Induction Phase

The induction phase can be broken into three steps. It is a good idea to keep these in mind as a guide in any method used to induce hypnosis. The first step is to describe to the subject the symptoms he *is about to* experience. The second step consists of suggestions of these symptoms, given in the *present tense,* as actually occurring. This is usually done in a gentle way using a relatively monotonous low tone of voice. The third step actually merges into the third phase (to be discussed later) and introduces it. As soon as there are indications the subject is hypnotized, the suggestions are given in a more *direct and emphatic* manner. These steps are particularly suited to the "sleep suggestion" method of inducing hypnosis, but apply with a few alterations to many other techniques. One exception is in the case of "instantaneous hypnosis" which we will talk about later.

Regardless of how the subject responded to the preparatory phase, tell him he can open his eyes again and to sit in the chair. In a conversational manner say to him:

I want you to look upward at a spot on the ceiling or the wall and to stare at that spot. Any spot will do, you can pick an imaginary spot if you wish. Pick a spot that is comfortable to fixate on. Don't be concerned if your eyes stray from the spot or you blink. If you do, just bring your eyes right back to the spot and continue to fixate on it the best you can. Just let yourself relax and listen closely to my voice, to what I say. I want you to relax...

Think of relaxing. Feel your body relaxing...As you think about relaxing, you will find your body relaxing...You will relax more and more. As you continue to look at the spot above your head and listen to my voice you will become aware that your entire body is becoming relaxed. Your feet are becoming relaxed, your legs are becoming relaxed, your arms and hands are becoming relaxed, your entire body is becoming relaxed. Now you will find that you are also becoming drowsy. You will become more and more drowsy. Just listen to my voice...it makes you feel drowsy, sleepy...You feel heaviness flowing all through your body. Your body is getting heavy, very h-e-a-v-y. Your arms are becoming h-e-a-v-y. Your hands and your arms are heavy. Your feet are getting h-e-a-v-y. Your entire body is becoming h-e-a-v-y, v-e-r-y h-e-a-v-y. You are d-r-o-w-s-y s-l-e-e-p-y. A pleasant feeling of drowsy warmth is coming over you. Soon you are going to sleep...deeply...soundly...A pleasant warmth is coming all over your body, just like when you fall asleep at night...Your eyes are getting heavy. You are becoming sleepy. Your eyes are getting heavier and h-e-a-v-i-e-r, s-o h-e-a-v-y. You are feeling s-o s-l-e-e-p-y.

Think of sleep, nothing but sleep...Very soon you are going to go to sleep...My voice makes you sleepy...makes you want to sleep...Your eye lids are heavy, they are closing. You cannot keep your eyes open. They are closing. Shortly you will find it impossible to keep your eyes open and they will begin to blink...They will blink more and more and in a moment they will close because they are getting heavier and heavier...you find it harder and harder to keep them open. [*You should try to coordinate this suggestion with the actual blinking of the subject's eyes. Some subjects are able to keep a steady unblinking stare and by giving the above suggestion they will often begin to blink. If they should not, it is best not to insist on this as it is not actually essential.*]

You are now v-e-r-y s-l-e-e-p-y...You eye lids are s-o h-e-a-v-y you cannot keep your eyes open. They are closing, closing more and more, more and more [*If you find the subject is not showing any indication of closing his eyes at this time, tell him in a firm voice:*] All right, now close your eyes and keep listening closely to what I say. [*Then continue with:*]

Your eyes are now closed and you are going deep asleep....[*Often a subject that has responded poorly to eye closure suggestions may develop some degree of hypnosis after closing his eyes. Also, some subjects pass into a relatively deep state of hypnosis quite early in the process but keep their eyes open and for some reason do not respond well to suggestions of eye closure. In any case, continue with:*] They are now closed and you are going into a deep sleep...a d-e-e-e-r and d-e-e-p-e-r sleep...You will pay attention to nothing but the sound of my voice. You will not awaking until I tell you to. Nothing will disturb you. Any time in the future I suggest sleep or say the word 'sleep' to you, you will instantly go into a deep sleep. You are now going to sleep deeply...v-e-r-y d-e-e-p-l-y. [*These last suggestions are important and should be given soon after the subject's eyes close. They should be restated a number of times. They will give you much better control over the subject than otherwise.*]

You can slightly vary the above procedure by standing close to the subject and raising your hand above the subjects head with the index and middle fingers spread apart in a V. Have the subject fixate on the fingers (rather than an imaginary spot). The suggestions you give are the same except if the subject appears to show some resistance to closing his eyes or is slow in doing so, continue by saying: "...your eyes are closing...closing, closing...*they are closed!*" As you say this bring your hand down rapidly toward the subject's face in such a way each of your two fingers come close to one eye. You can stop with out touching the subject's eyes, or you can stop and press gently on the subject's closed eyes to emphasize your statement of closure. Of course, by bringing your fingers so near to the subject's eyes in a sudden manner you force him to close them by a reflex action. For your first few inductions of hypnosis you should not attempt to do more than this.

When giving the above suggestions you should generally speak in a quite monotone. However, you will find it helpful to make use of inflections and other effects from time to time, some of which we have tried to indicate. When suggesting that the eyes are closing, and you can see some response is occurring, it is often helpful to quicken your speech, raise your voice somewhat, add some excitement to it, and repeat the suggestion over and over rapidly. This suggests to the subject that something is really happening. A decisive "*They are closed!*" will often over come any remaining tendency of the subject to keep his eyes open. However, some subjects may never completely close their eyes. You may be able to see the white of the eyes through a small slit. Also the eyelids may show a rapid trembling that may give the appearance that the subject is resisting or about to open his eyes. Actually these subjects may be very deeply hypnotized.

Lets stop here for a moment and talk about what a hypnotized person looks like. The typical and traditional picture of a hypnotized person usually found in books and magazines is that of an individual who appears to be fast asleep or in a dead faint. It is true that subjects often appear to be soundly asleep by the time the induction phase is completed. Their eyes are closed, the muscles of the face are relaxed, and their entire body is quite relaxed. If he is sitting in a chair, he will often be slumped down in it. His head often falls forward on his chest, or backward or sometimes sideways on his shoulder. His arms and hands usually rest limply by his sides. The onset of this condition may occur very gradually, or it may suddenly and rapidly appear.

Unfortunately, the above description fails to materialize in many cases. An appreciable number of subjects do not show these characteristics, evenly if deeply hypnotized. These characteristics are not necessarily a criterion of deep hypnosis. Muscular relaxation is not an essential correlate of hypnosis. Many subjects remain upright when hypnotized while sitting. They may also show considerable stiffness, and even an unusual amount of rigidity. Even eye closure is not an essential criterion or requirement for hypnosis.

There are some characteristics that generally do distinguish the hypnotized person from a non-hypnotized person. The most characteristic symptom immediately following the induction of hypnosis is a tendency toward *protracted immobility*. The subject may be relaxed or tense, his eyes open or closed, he may be comfortable or uncomfortable, but nearly always, if not always, he displays an amazing degree of immobility, unless suggestions are given calling for movement. Some subjects may show spontaneous movements, but they are very limited in duration and are probably do to a reflex. There is usually a lack of facial expression. If the eyes are open, the gaze is fixed and blank.

Subjects have a strong *disinclination to speak*. It is often necessary to address them several times before obtaining an answer. On occasion it may be necessary to order them to answer questions. Even then most subjects will nod or shake their head rather than speak. When some sort of conversation has been established, subjects usually lack spontaneity and initiative. Their speech tends to be low in volume, flat and expressionless. They tend to mumble their answers and must be ordered to speak louder and more distinctly. If motor responses are elicited, they tend to be overly slow and stiff. *Psychomotor retardation* is often present and also a degree of *automatism*.

The above description best describes hypnotized individuals immediately following the appearance of hypnosis. As subjects are made to carry out an increasing number of suggestions, the characteristics described above tend to decrease in intensity and even vanish. In many cases there are few or no symptoms that can be used to distinguish the hypnotized subject from a person in the normal waking state. However, even when most hypnotized individuals are acting in a normal way, there still tends to be a constriction of awareness, a characteristic literal-mindedness, some psychomotor retardation and a small degree of automatism. There also is usually a relative lack of humor or self-consciousness.

The demeanor of a subject following the induction of hypnosis is partly do to the manner in which hypnosis was induced and the subject's expectations. An individual that is hypnotized while standing up is going to show less relaxation than an individual that was hypnotized sitting down or reclining. However, on occasion you might encounter a subject whose concept of hypnosis, as a state of complete relaxation, is so strong that when hypnotized in the standing position he will collapse to the floor. Even with sitting subjects, the initial conditions at the beginning of the induction may prevent a relaxed state from occurring. Individuals who for one reason or another tense all or part of their body at the beginning of the induction often retain this condition. The subject's expectation or concept of hypnosis can play a large part in how he reacts to hypnosis. If he expects to be physically relaxed, relaxation is most likely to be a symptom of hypnosis in his case. However, if he expects to behave like a zombie, this is the type of behavior you are apt to see. The type of instructions given to the subject, the manner they are given, and his own interpretation of them, are strong determinants in the way he will behave when hypnotized.

The best criterion, by far, of hypnosis is *hyper-suggestibility*. However, this is much more an indicator of the depth of hypnosis the subject has obtained rather than an absolute indicator of the presence or absence of hypnosis.

Deepening The Trance

As soon as the subject's eyes close, you are ready to deepen the trance. At this point the depth of trance could be anywhere from a very light one to a very deep one. For our purposes we will assume it is moderately deep (it usually is). The deepening process generally consists of giving suggestions that:

1. The trance is getting progressively deeper

2. Allow periods of silence

3. Ask for a variety of graded responses

In addition in a later module we will introduce special techniques for deepening the trance.

The first technique listed above, is fairly obvious. The second is best employed following suggestions of deeper hypnosis. The periods of silence can last from a few seconds to 30 minutes. The suggestions to initiate a period of silence can be of the form of: "In a moment I will stop talking to you for a while. You will continue to sleep deeply. In fact, you will keep going deeper and deeper asleep. When I talk to you again, you will much deeper asleep...much more than now. You feel very comfortable and nothing will disturb you. You will not awaken until I tell you to. When I next speak to you, you will not be startled by my voice. Now I will stop talking to you, but you will continue to go deeper and deeper asleep." Many hypnotists believe that periods of silence allow suggestions to take full effect and allow the hypnotic state to develop more fully. Presumably the processes involved in the induction of hypnosis or the responses to suggestions are not instantaneous. There is some evidence that indicates a radical change in neural activity takes place not only when trance-inducing suggestions are given, put when any suggestion is given.

How long should the period of silence be? I don't have a good answer to this. If the period is too long, there is the danger the subject may pass into a state of natural sleep -- he then is no longer hypnotized. The frequency and length you will just have to learn by experience.

The last procedure listed, consists of giving the subject a series of graded suggestions. When a subject carries out a variety of suggestions, he usually appears to become increasingly responsive. There is no reason to believe that the processes used to produce the hypnotic state stop when eye closure is achieved. To the contrary, there is considerable evidence that eye closure can be brought about with a relative small amount of suggestibility. Much less than the subject's potential. This is the rational for continuing what was done in the preparatory phase and induction phase. As emphasized earlier, the use of graded suggestions is important in order to avoid creating negative attitudes through failure to respond adequately, and to trigger homoaction and heteroaction.

Most hypnotists follow eye closure with suggested eye catalepsy, with out the instructions to turn the eyes upward. If you have been successful in obtaining eye catalepsy in the waking state, or if you are confident the subject is sufficiently hypnotized, you can end this suggestion with the usual challenge. However, if there is any doubt about the outcome, it is best not to challenge the subject because the trance could be broken if the subject is able to open his eyes. Although the rejection of a suggestion does not necessarily mean the state of hypnosis has ended, a good rule to follow is when in doubt about the success of any hypnotic suggestion, you should not challenge the subject to overcome it. Instead, try to deepen the trance.

If you decide not to challenge the eye catalepsy, you have two choices. You can say nothing about attempts to open the eyes, but go to the next suggest. The second choice is to say something like this: "Your eyelids are stuck tightly together...so tight that *if* you tried to open them *you could not*. But you will *not* try to open them. *You have no desire* to open them, you only want to sleep."

The next suggestion that is usually given is arm rigidity. Some hypnotists give it before eye catalepsy, or instead of it. Arm rigidity is one suggestion that should always be challenged. If a subject is not hypnotized deeply enough to make this suggestion effective, you might as well start hypnotizing him all over again, using a different method.

The following is a sample procedure for deepening the trance. It should be made continuous with the suggestions of the induction phase. It should be given immediately after eye closure:

Sleep...deeply...very deeply. Your eyelids are heavy...v-e-r-y h-e-a-v-y...They are stuck tight, so tightly stuck that you cannot open them no matter how hard you try. YOU CANNOT OPEN YOUR EYES. TRY! YOU CANNOT OPEN THEM...try hard...All right now, stop trying. You are going deeper asleep...much deeper. Lift your arm up [*as you say this take hold of the subject's hand and gently guide his hand and arm straight out to the side at shoulder height.*]

Extend it straight out. Make a fist...a tight fist...TIGHTER! Your arm is stiffening; your entire arm is becoming stiff! STIFF! RIGID! LIKE A BAR OF STEEL! YOU CANNOT BEND YOUR ARM, YOU CANNOT MOVE IT. Try. YOU CAN'T...*try hard*...All right now, you can move it. [*With some individuals you may have to give more counter suggestions than this.* Slowly lower it to your lap. As you do you will go deeper and deeper asleep...d-e-e-p-e-r and d-e-e-p-e-r. You are now deeply asleep. S-l-e-e-p! D-e-e-p, d-e-e-p asleep!...Your entire body is now very relaxed.

You have no desire to move. You only wish to s-l-e-e-p...d-e-e-p-l-y...s-o-u-n-d-l-y...You want to do what ever I ask you to do. You can hear me clearly. You will be able to answer my questions and do everything I ask you to do, but you will remain deep asleep. If I tell you to open your eyes, you will not awaken until I tell you to. Any time in the future I tell you to sleep you will *immediately* go into a very deep sleep. As soon as I say 'sleep' your eyelids will get very heavy, you will get very sleepy, your eyes will close, you will go deeply asleep...This will happen each and every time I say the word 'sleep.' [*You can if you wish substitute at this point some other signal, or add to the above instruction. We will have more to say about this later*]

Now just continue sleeping...d-e-e-p-l-y, s-o-u-n-d-l-y...I am going to stop talking to you for a short time, but you will continue to go deeper asleep. Nothing will disturb you...you will only hear the sound of my voice. When I speak to you again you will not be startled...Now sleep...d-e-e-p-l-y. [*Stop talk talking for 5 to 15 minutes, then in a very low voice (even a whisper), continue your suggestions. Gradually but fairly rapidly increase the volume of your voice.*] You are now deep asleep. You can hear everything clearly, but you will only pay attention to the sound of my voice. [*You said earlier the subject would only hear the sound of your voice. With a very suggestible subject this may have the effect of making him deaf to all other sounds. You must be careful to remove this condition, if it exists.*]

Unless you want to deepen the trance more, you should give the subject more complex suggestions in order to determine his depth of hypnosis. If you prefer you can wake your subject up without further testing. But we will assume that you test him and find he is not as deeply hypnotized as you want. This being the case you can continue by saying to the subject:

You are deep asleep, but you can go even more deeply asleep than you are now. It is your desire to sleep as deeply as possible because it is a very pleasant experience, and it is of great benefit to you. You are going to sleep much more deeply and will respond positively to all the suggestions I give you. I shall now count to three [*You can use any number you want here*] and as I do you will begin to drift down into a much deeper sleep, and at the count of three you will be very, very sound asleep. So sound asleep that when I ask you to awaken later [*It is preferable to say "when I ask you to awaken" rather than "when you awaken" because the former reinforces the contingency of waking upon your command, where the later does not and could be interpreted by the subject as giving him some control over the matter of waking.*] you will have no memory of anything that was said or done while you were asleep. It will be as though no time had passed and you had not slept.

I will now start counting. One..You are going deeply, much more d-e-e-p-l-y asleep. Two..you are going d-e-e-p-e-r and d-e-e-p-e-r asleep. With each count you go deeper asleep. With each word I say you go deeper asleep. With each easy breath you take you go deeper asleep. You can feel yourself drifting down into a very pleasant deep sleep. [*At this point you can begin to soften and lower your voice.*] You can feel yourself drifting deeper and deeper asleep. You hear nothing but the sound of my voice. The sound of my voice makes you sleepy. My voice sounds as though it were coming from far away. All the suggestions I give you in the future will be effective. You will do everything I ask you to do. As I continue to talk to you go deeper asleep. Any time I tell you to see, hear, smell or feel something you will see, hear, smell or feel it. What I suggest will become reality. You will experience it fully. Every time in the future that I tell you to do something when you are hypnotized, and only then, [*This provision is added to eliminate the possibility that the subject will post hypnotically become dominated by the hypnotist. This is a matter of ethics as well as a safeguard for both the hypnotist and subject.*] you will carry it out without question...I will always be able to remove and change any suggestion that I give you now, have given you, or will have given you. [*This is extremely important and this suggestion should always be given and repeated a number of times. Now allow a few moments of silence.*]...Continue to sleep. At the next count you will be deeply, soundly asleep. [*Allow another period of silence here.*] Three... Deep, d-e-e-p asleep! You will not awaken until I tell

69

you to or unless something should happen to me or something occurs that demands your attention. Otherwise you will remain deep asleep and will do everything I ask you to do. Anytime in the future I say sleep or suggest sleep [*include another signal (i.e., snap of my fingers) here if you have given one.*] you will *instantly*, go into a deep sleep, even deeper than you are now. When I awaken you later you will have no memory of anything but having slept.

At this point you are ready to use the hypnotic trance for whatever purpose you have created it for.

With passive subjects the above technique may cause them to go into a lethargic or stuporous state that is difficult to alter. Because they are already prone to passivity, it is probably best to make use of procedures for deepening the trance which de-emphasize passivity and maximize the use of activity. It is especially inadvisable to suggest to such subjects a desire for sleep, or that sleep is a desirable state. Instead suggestions to deepening the trance should emphasize a desire for activity and cooperation. The technique of fractionation that will be taken up in another module is particularly suited here.

"Waking" The Subject

Normally waking up the subject, or more precisely his *de-hypnotization*, is one of the simplest parts of hypnotism. Generally it is only necessary to order the subject, "Wake up!" in a firm but gentle voice. Or you could say: "When I snap my fingers and tell you to wake up, you will be wide awake, feeling wonderful in every way." This is followed by snapping your fingers and the command "Wake up!" For subjects that have been in a deep trance, this form of de-hypnotizing may be a little brusque or unpleasant, especially if they have been in a passive state for some time. In this case it is better to make the process gentle and gradual. One-way to do this is as follows: "In a moment you are going to slowly awaken. I will count from one up to five; at the count of five, you will be wide-awake, feeling wonderful in every way. Now I am beginning to count. One...you are going to awaking very soon...Two...you are slowly beginning to awaken...Three..you are becoming more awake...Four...at the next count you will be wide awaking, feeling perfect in every way...*Five...Wide-awake!* You are alert, feeling better than you have ever felt before. Take a deep breath, and relax."

On occasion, when the subject opens his eyes after being awakened he appears somewhat dazed. If asked to stand up he may seem unsteady on his legs. This usually indicates that the subject is not fully de-hypnotized. It may be the result of awaking the subject too quickly. In such a case you should take additional measures to completely awaken the subject. One way is to snap your fingers near the subjects face and say in a firm voice *"Wake up! Wide awake!"* In awaking the subject, there is one rule that should always be followed: **Never allow a subject to leave you until you have made certain he is fully de-hypnotized, no matter how light his trance may have been.** It is a good idea to have the subject sit nearby for a short time so you can observe him. Before letting him leave ask him a few questions about how he is feeling.

A Quick Method of Induction

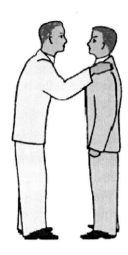

Figure 10-1

Have your subject stand in front of you and place your hands on his shoulders. Bring your face close to his, approximately 8 or 9 inches away and fixate on the bridge of his nose (See Figure 10-1). Say to the subject: "Look into my eyes and think of sleep. You are going to go to sleep, quickly, deeply...You are going into a deep sound sleep. Keep looking into my eyes. As you do you feel a heaviness coming over your body...Your body is getting heavy...Your legs are heavy, very heavy. Your arms are heavy, very heavy. Your hands and arms are heavy as lead. Your entire body is heavy...s-o h-e-a-v-y. Your eyelids are getting heavy...you are getting sleepy...drowsy...You are tired...your body is so heavy...You want to sleep. Your eyelids are so heavy you cannot keep them open. They are closing...closing...closing...You cannot keep them open...You're going to sleep...Your eyes are closed, *Sleep!* DEEP ASLEEP!

Another Rapid Method of Inducing Hypnosis

This method is ideal when you want to combine testing for hypnotic susceptibility with the induction of hypnosis. Proceed rapidly through the postural sway, hand clasping, and eye catalepsy suggestions in the order given. If the subject gives good strong responses to each of the above, then as soon as you are satisfied he cannot open his eyes, instead of telling him he can open them, proceed as follows:

All right now, stop trying to open your eyes. You are now going to go to sleep. Sleep!...DEEP ASLEEP! [*Following the eye catalepsy suggestions, move your hand downward in front of the subject's face, form a V with the index and middle finger and gently press the subject's closed eyes for a brief moment. Then place your hands on the subject's shoulders. All of this should take only a moment without any obvious break in the suggestions. In many cases the subject will be in a relative deep trance, but it is best to carry the induction a little farther before testing for depth. You can consider the remainder of this procedure as part of the induction proper, or as part of the deepening phase. With your hands lightly grasp the subject's shoulders and very gently move his body in a slight rotary motion using his feet as a pivot point. At the same time continue giving more suggestions.*] You are now drifting into a deep...d-e-e-p sleep. You will not awaken until I tell you to...waves of sleep are coming over you...you are going deeper and deeper asleep. Your body feels heavy...your hands and arms are heavy, v-e-r-y heavy...Your feet and legs are s-o h-e-av-y. You feel yourself drifting into a deep sound sleep. Sleep...deeply...soundly...S-l-e-e-p. [*At this time take hold of his forearm, raise it horizontally to his side saying at the same time:*] Now raise your arm...Make a tight fist. [*Give the arm rigidity suggestions for deepening the trance as was done in the first method. After the challenge, ask the subject to lower his arm slowly, guiding it if necessary, and suggest the trance is getting deeper. As soon as his arm is by his side, continue as follows:*] You are now deep asleep and going even deeper asleep...Take a deep breath...breath deeply and slowly...with each breath you take you go deeper and deeper asleep. Continue to breathe deeply...Sleep...You only desire to sleep. You only think of sleep. Breathe deeply...Sleep deeply...More and more deeply...Each and every time in the future that I tell you to sleep, suggest sleep, or say the word 'sleep' you will instantly go into a deep, sound sleep. Even deeper asleep than now. You will remain asleep until I tell you to awaken or until something happens that demands your attention. You will remain deep asleep. Nothing will bother you. Listen to only the sound of my voice.

Comments on Methods

In this module you have been given three methods of inducing hypnosis. Before trying any of the methods presented in the following modules, *you should make every effort to master the procedures in this module.* These three procedures embody most of the elements that are used in any technique.

As you are probably aware, you have done nothing here that differs essentially from what you did in working with waking suggestions. The initial portion of the induction involves waking suggestions. Certain procedural features appear to run through all modern trance-inducing techniques. For example, a combination of attention focusing (usually involving visual and auditory fixation) with suggestions of some of the superficial symptoms of the appearance of sleep and of sleep itself, ending in suggested eye closure. However, introducing the concept of sleep and its symptoms is not always necessary. But so far we have been talking about the Standard method of inducing hypnosis. We will end this module with the following general rules:

1. If it is not necessary to obtain a deep trance, a rapid induction will probably be satisfactory. But, if a deep trance is required, then it is best to use a slower method.

2. A rapid method will impress an audience more than a slow one. If you have access to a fair number of subjects you can enhance the effectiveness of a demonstration by using a rapid method, even though deep hypnosis will not be induced in all the subjects.

3. Failure to induce hypnosis by one method can hinder subsequent attempts to induce a trance by other methods. Because the likelihood of failure is greater with rapid methods, it is best to use slower methods where the number of subjects is limited.

4. For experimental and therapeutic purposes the slow methods are usually preferred because they allow greater control over the trance and there is a greater chance of success. However, some subjects only respond well to certain techniques that are considered rapid techniques.

MODULE 11 -- INDUCTION OF HYPNOSIS

Advanced Techniques

Most of the innumerable induction techniques are virtually variations of the procedures we have already practiced. It would be impractical to discuss all of them and it is not necessary. There are a small number that are worth describing fully. Others of lesser value we will briefly outline. It is a good idea to try each of the methods presented in this module. The order in which you try them is unimportant, but you should master them completely in order to use them effectively.

Hand Levitation Method

This procedure was first described by M. H. Erickson, however, one of the best descriptions of it was given by L. R. Wolberg. He had this to say about the procedure: "I believe this is the best of all induction procedures. It permits of a participation in the induction process by the patient and lends itself to non-directive and analytic techniques. It is, however, the most difficult of methods and calls for greater endurance on the part of the hypnotist."

Wolberg started with a brief preparatory phase and continued as follows (The suggestions are a verbatim report of a recorded induction session):

I want you to sit comfortably in your chair and relax. As you sit there, bring both hands palms down on your thigh -- just like that. Keep watching your hands, and you will notice that you are able to observe them closely.

What you will do is sit in the chair and relax. Then you will notice certain things happen in the course of relaxing. They always have happened while relaxing, but you have not noticed them so closely before. I am going to point them out to you. I'd like you to concentrate on all sensations and feelings in your hands no matter what they may be. Perhaps you may feel the heaviness of your hand as it lies on your thigh, or you may feel pressure. Perhaps you will feel the texture of your trousers as they press against the palm of your hand; or the warmth of your hand on your thigh. Perhaps you may feel tingling. No matter what sensations there are, I want you to observe them. Keep watching your hand, and you will notice how quite it is, how it remains in one position. There is motion there, but it is not yet noticeable. I want you to keep watching your hand. Your attention may wander from the hand, but it will always return back to the hand, and you keep watching the hand and wondering when the motion that is there will show itself.

At this point the patient's attention is fixed on his hand. He is curious about what will happen, and sensations such as any person might experience are suggested to him as possibilities. No attempt is being made to force any suggestions on him, and if he observes any sensations or feelings, he incorporates them as a product of his own experience. The object eventually is to get him to respond to the suggestions of the hypnotist as if these too are a part of his own experiences. A subtle attempt is being made to get him to associate his sensations with the words spoken to him so that the words or commands uttered by the hypnotist will evoke sensory or motor responses later on. Unless the patient is consciously resisting, a slight motion or jerking will develop in one of the fingers or in the hand. As soon as this happens, the hypnotist mentions it and remarks that the motion will probably increase. The hypnotist must also comment on any other objective reaction of the patient, such as motion of the legs or deep breathing. The result of this linking of the patient's reactions with comments of the hypnotist is an association of the two in the patient's mind.

It will be interesting to see which one of the fingers will move first. It may be the middle finger, or the forefinger, or the ring finger, or the thumb. One of the fingers is going to jerk or move. You don't know exactly when or in which hand. Keep watching and you will notice a slight movement, possible in the right hand. There, the thumb jerks and moves, just like that.

As the movement begins you will notice an interesting thing. Very slowly the spaces between the fingers will widen, the fingers will slowly move apart, and you'll notice that the spaces will get wider and wider and wider. They'll move apart slowly; the fingers will seem to be spreading apart, wider and wider and wider. The fingers are spreading, wider and wider apart, just like that.

This is the first real suggestion to which the patient is expected to respond. If the fingers start spreading apart, they do so because the patient is reacting to suggestion. The hypnotist continues to talk as if the response is one that could have come about by itself in the natural course if events.

As the fingers spread apart, you will notice that the fingers will soon want to arch up from the thigh, as if they wanted to lift, higher and higher. [*The patient's index finger starts moving upward slightly.*] Notice how the index finger lifts. As it does the other fingers want to follow -- up, up, slowly rising. [*The other fingers start lifting.*]

As the fingers lift you will notice a lightness in the hand. A feeling of lightness, so much so that the fingers will arch up, and the whole hand will slowly lift and rise as if it feels like a feather, as a balloon is lifting it up in the air, lifting. Lifting, -- up--up--up, pulling up higher and higher and higher, the hand is becoming very light. [*The hand starts rising.*] As you watch your hand rise, you'll notice that the arm comes up, up, up in the air, a little higher -- and higher -- and higher -- and higher, up -- up -- up. [*The arm has lifted about five inches above the thigh and the patient is gazing at it fixedly.*]

Keep watching the hand and arm as it rises straight up, and as it does you will soon become aware of how drowsy and tired your eyes become. As your arm continues to rise, you will get tired and relaxed and sleepy, very sleepy. Your eyes will get heavy and your lids may want to close. And as your arm rises higher and higher, you will want to feel more relaxed and sleepy, and you will want to enjoy the peaceful relaxed feeling of letting your eyes close and of being sleepy.

[*It will be noted that as the patient executes one suggestion, his positive response is used to reinforce the next suggestion. For instance, as his arm rises, it is suggested in essence that he will get drowsy because his arm is rising.*]

Your arm lifts -- up -- up -- and you are getting very drowsy; your lids get very heavy, your breathing gets slow and regular. Breathe deeply -- in and out. [*The patient holds his arm stretched out directly in front of him, his eyes are blinking and his breathing is deep and regular.*] As you keep watching your hand and arm and feeling more and more drowsy and relaxed, you will notice that the direction of the hand will change. The arm will bend, and the hand will move closer and closer to your face -- up -- up -- up and as it rises you will slowly but steadily go into a deep, deep, sleep in which you relax deeply and to your satisfaction. The arm will continue to rise up -- up -- lifting, lifting, -- up in the air until it touches your face, and you will get sleeper and sleeper, but you must not go to sleep until your hand touches your face. When your hand touches your face you will be asleep, deeply asleep.

The patient here is requested to choose his own pace in falling asleep, so that when his hand touches his face, he feels himself to be asleep to his own satisfaction. Hand levitation and sleepiness continue to reinforce each other. When the patient finally does close his eyes, he will have entered a trance with his own participation. He will later be less inclined to deny that he has been in a trance.

Your hand is now changing its direction. It moves up -- up -- up -- up toward your face. Your eyelids are getting heavy. You are getting sleeper, and sleeper, and sleeper. [*The patient's hand is approaching his face, his eyelids are blinking more rapidly.*] Your eyes get heavy, very heavy, and your hand moves straight up toward your face. You get very tired and drowsy. Your eyes are closing, are closing. When your hand touches your face you'll be asleep, deeply asleep. You feel very drowsy. You feel drowsier and drowsier and drowsier, very sleepy, very tired. Your eyes are like lead, and your hand moves up, up, up, right toward your face, and when it touches your face, you will be asleep. [*Patient's hand touches his face and his eyes close.*] Go to sleep, go to sleep, just sleep. And as you sleep you feel very tired and relaxed. I want you to concentrate on relaxation, a state of tensionless relaxation. Think of nothing else, but sleep, deep sleep.

H. Arons described an interesting variation of the Wolberg technique that tends to be more rapid (probably at a cost of the percentage of successes and depth of trance). The subject is instructed to stand facing the hypnotist, stretch out his right arm and point at the hypnotist's feet while fixing his gaze on his pointing finger.

These instructions are followed by suggestions that his arm will become light and his arm will rise. He is told that his arm will rise upward toward the hypnotist's eyes and that the subject's eyes will remain focused on his finger as his arm rises. The hypnotist continues to suggest that the subject's hand will rise until his finger points at the hypnotist's eyes and when this occurs their gaze will meet. The subject is told that as soon as this happens he will instantly fall into a deep hypnotic sleep. When the subject begins to show some response to this suggestion, the hypnotist should change his suggestions accordingly. As soon as the subject's finger points at the hypnotist's eyes and their gazes meet the hypnotist should forcefully command the subject to sleep.

Folding Hand Method

F. F. Wagner first described this method. He found that it was sometimes difficult to get the subject's hand up to his face using Wolberg's technique. This was mainly do to mechanical factors and because the abnormal protracted position of the hands may become painfully tiring for some subjects. He modified the procedure so that the last phase of the trance induction is replaced by hand clasping. In this way only the forearms and hands are involved. Wagner described it as follows:

In short the method is as follows: After careful preparation, hypnosis commences as in the hand levitation method. The initial position is the same (see Figure 11-1A). First, the fingers of one hand are

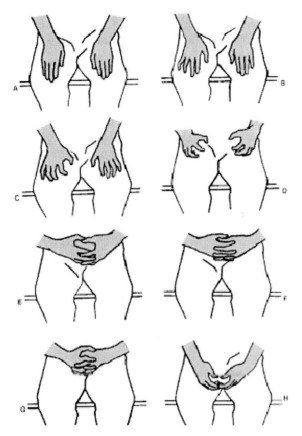

induced to spread out (Fig. 11-1B); secondly, the flexing of the fingers and simultaneously spreading of the fingers of the other hand. When both hands have been raised from the thigh (Fig. 11-1C), suggestions are given that the palms will turn to each other (Fig. 11-1D); and that they will be attracted to each other like opposite poles of a magnet (Fig. 11-1E). Gradually as the hands get closer together, general suggestions are given of increasing drowsiness, deeper breathing and sensations of heaviness of the eyelids. These suggestions are enforced while the fingers interlace (Fig. 11-1F). The hands are clinched simultaneously with eyelids drooping. When the clinching of the hands reaches its maximum (Fig.11-1G), general relaxation and heaviness of the whole body including arms and eyelids is suggested; the hands slip apart (Fig. 11-1H). Then the trance may be deepened in the usual manner, or the patient may be wakened if a fractional technique is preferred.

FIG. 11-1

Wagner states that most people get a very intense feeling of mutual attraction of the hands. This, he says, considerably intensifies the suggestibility. He also states that anxiety that may be aroused during the hypnotic session tends to dissipate as soon as the hands are folded.

Postural Sway Methods

This can be an extraordinarily rapid method of inducing hypnosis. It can be applied when a subject responds well to the postural sway test of suggestibility. The follow procedure is a verbatim report of this procedure by J. G. Watkins:

The therapist speaks to the patient as follows: "Now Jones, I'd like you to stand here with your heels and your toes together and your body erect, shoulders back. That's right. Breathe comfortably and easily with your hands at your sides. Now close your eyes. Just imagine that your feet are hinged to the floor and your body is like a stick pointing upward in the air, free to move back and forth. You will probably feel after a while, you will become unsteady. Don't worry, if you should fall, I'll catch you." *[This last remark is given in a matter-of-fact way, almost as a side comment. If previous suggestibility tests have been given, and the therapist is quite certain the patient will enter the trance, he may modify this statement by saying, "Don't worry, I will catch you when you fall."]*

The therapist then continues: "Now while you are standing there, breathe very calmly and easily. Just imagine that your body is floating up into space. Don't try to do anything, and don't try *not* to do anything. Just stand there and let yourself drift. " The therapist is then silent for a time, perhaps fifteen seconds up to a minute. If the patient is suggestible he will sway back and forth slightly.

The therapist should place himself at the side of the patient where he can line the back of the patient's head or the tip of his nose against a mark on the opposite wall so that a slight backward or forward swaying movement can be easily detected and measured. It is even convenient to have a card against the wall on which black vertical lines have been ruled about an inch apart, thus making it easier to determine the amount of sway. Usually the therapist will soon detect the rhythm of the swaying, since it is almost impossible for anybody to stand perfectly still. There will always be some swaying, although it may be slight in the more unsuggestible patients. One will generally find that the more suggestible the patient, the greater will be the amplitude of the swaying arc.

The therapist next begins to reinforce this swaying by timing his remarks to coincide with it. As soon as the patient has reached the extreme forward part of the arc and begins to sway backward the therapist says, "Now you are drifting backward." Frequently this will cause the patient to immediately catch himself and to reverse the direction, whereupon the therapist instantly reinforces it with, "Now you are drifting forward." As the swaying continues the therapist reinforces it with "Drifting forward, drifting backward and forward, backward, forward, backward," etc. The tone is low, soft, and firm. The therapist should be about one to two feet away from the patient's ear and should repeat the suggestions in a low, soft monotone from which all harshness has been deleted. It should have an almost pleasing quality, monotonous like the drone of a bee. There should be no change in pitch, and the patter should be continued steadily. Occasionally it may be varied from "drifting forward" to "swaying forward, swaying backward, swaying forward, now swaying forward." or "leaning forward, backward, forward, backward." etc. -- on and on in a monotonous, repetitious voice.

As the therapist observes the amplitude of the swaying arc increasing, he may make the voice somewhat less pleading, less soft, and more dominant and controlling, even injecting some emotional pitch into the "forward, backward, forward, backward."

When the amplitude of the swaying arc has become quite substantial -- six or more inches -- it is probable that some light degree of trance has been induced (note that the suggestions of sleep do not come up until quite late in this procedure.). Suggestibility should then be checked by beginning a command of "forward, backward" a little before the patient has reached the maximum sway of the arc. If the patient is suggestible, and there is a degree of hypnotic trance, he will interrupt the natural sway in order to follow the therapist's suggestions. The past remarks of the therapist have so closely followed the patient's swaying behavior that the patient begins to think to himself, "What this man says is true, I am swaying backward. Then I do sway forward." Consequently, the therapist's prestige is increased, and the patient begins to follow the suggestions instead of leading them. From this point on the therapist can usually assume the more dominating role and direct rather than follow the swaying of the patient.

To induce deeper trance the voice tone is now made much firmer and the swaying suggestions are given somewhat more rapidly. "*Swaying forward, swaying backward, forward, backward,*" the volume of the voice growing stronger and stronger. Finally, an attempt is made to induce the patient to fall over backward into a deep trance. The emphasis on the "backward" is increased, and on the "forward" diminished, and the verb is changed from "drifting" or "swaying" to "Falling, *falling backward,* falling forward, *falling backward*, falling forward, *falling over backward,* falling, falling, *falling, falling"* rather rapidly and in a higher pitched and more emotional tone. If a deep trance has been induced, the patient will increase the amplitude of his away until he can no longer stand erect. He will then fall over backward in a deep trance where he may be caught by the therapist and eased into a waiting chair.

If the patient is in a light trance he may start to fall backward, but catch himself by placing one of his feet back, or attempt to sway sideways or steady himself voluntarily in some manner. This indicates to the therapist that a deep trance has not been induced and he can then do one of two things: he may either continue the monotonous repetition of "falling forward, falling backward," etc., to induce a deeper degree of trance; or he may reassure the patient that he will not fall by placing a hand lightly behind his shoulder. This allays fears that might arise and interrupts the hypnotic process. After the patient realizes that he will not be permitted to fall and hurt himself, he tends to lose the signs of anxiety which may have begun to appear.. He may then allow himself to fall back against the therapist's arm, whereupon the therapist continues suggestions, "Falling over backward, falling backward, falling back into a deep sleep, back into a deep sleep, deep sleep, deep sleep," and then eases the patient gradually over into a chair. This, preferably an armchair, should have been placed behind the patient. He can also be gradually lowered back upon a couch that has been located conveniently near by.

If the patient is either completely limp or in a stiff catatonic state when he is placed back on the chair or cot, it is evident that a fairly deep degree of trance has been induced. If, however, he is able to help himself either by taking steps backward or by putting his hands on the arm chair and guiding himself into it, then only a light hypnoidal trance has been induced.

Watkins claims there are several advantages to this technique: It appears inoffensive to the subject, particularly since the hypnotist may present the procedure as a test of reflexes, etc. Because the method is not generally known to the public its use is not likely to cause anxiety or apprehension, as do the standard techniques.

The following method can be used to induce a trance, but it is given here primarily as an effective way of deepening the trance state. Watkins gives two variations that follow.

Metronome Method

Place a metronome, out of sight, near the subject. Watkins recommends setting the metronome to fifty beats per minute. He also suggests that the sound of the metronome be muffled by enclosing it in a box or cabinet. We now assume that the first phase of trance induction has been completed. At this point Watkins says:

He [the patient or subject] is told, "Now I am going to turn on a slow ticking sound. This will help you to go to sleep. Listen very carefully to it and to nothing else. It goes like this." The metronome is turned on. Then the therapist continues, "Just imagine each tick saying to you, 'deep -- sleep -- deep -- sleep,' and the deeper you go into sleep the deeper you will want to go. How comfortable you will feel all over. Just keep on listing to this ticking sound that says over and over again, 'deep -- sleep -- deep -- sleep.' The therapist may even continue speaking the words 'deep -- sleep' for a little while, while timing them to coincide with the ticking.

78

A second variation given by Watkins is:

Suggest to the patient that as he listens to the ticking he will imagine himself slowly going down a ladder or stairway. "Each tick is saying "step -- down, -- step -- down," or "deep -- sleep, -- step -- down," etc. He may be told, "As you go down this ladder you will feel that you are going down into a deeper and deeper sleep."

After a few moments Watkins leaves the subject, allowing him to listen to the metronome for 10 to 30 minutes. He also outlined a number of other minor variations. In one he tell the subject that he is going to leave him for a short time while the subject listens to the ticking, and that when he comes back he will be in the deepest possible sleep. The subject may also be told that when he reaches the deepest sleep, his hand will slowly rise and touch his forehead. The hypnotist checks periodically to observe whether this has taken place. Watkins points out that the use of the metronome, coupled with the above suggestions, is less fatiguing for the hypnotist.

Fractionation Method

O. Vogt was the first to describe this method. It is probably one of the most effective methods for inducing a very deep trance state, and often succeeds when every other method has failed. It is especially indicated if you expect your subject to enter, at best, a light or medium trance. It also is an effective method for handling subjects, who at first only experience a light state of hypnosis, and doubt that they have been hypnotized. Essentially, the method consists of hypnotizing and waking the subject in rapid consecutive successions. The idea is that each hypnotization makes the subject a little more suggestible and favors the induction of deeper hypnosis on the next trial. Substantial evidence indicates that the hypnotic state continues a short time after the subject is awakened, particularly if the awaking process is sudden.

An effective use of this technique is as follow: When you are ready to awaken the subject tell him the following: "In a moment I will tell you to awaken. When I do you will awake, but you will immediately feel very sleepy again. You will find it difficult to keep your eyes open and stay awake. Your eyelids will feel very heavy, and they will get heavier and heavier until you will not be able to keep them open any longer. You will not be able to prevent yourself from blinking and closing them. You will get sleepier and drowsier with each breath you take and in a moment your eyes will close. You will go deeply asleep, deeper than ever before. I will now count to three, at the count of three you will be awake and will open your eyes. But you will be drowsy and sleepy. Your eyes will be so heavy that you will not be able to keep them open very long, and will go back to sleep...Now, one...two...three...*Awake!*" As a rule the subject will remain sitting rather passively. He may start to blink or appear sleepy with his eyes have closed. Ask him what is the matter with his eyes. He may tell you he feels sleepy, but more often he will appear puzzled and say he doesn't know what the trouble is. In any case, continue by saying: "You feel kind of sleepy, don't you? It is difficult to keep your eyes open. [*At this point the subject almost always starts blinking before closing his eyes. Whatever he does you should make an effort to follow it up and incorporate it your next suggestions, which might be:*] Your eyes are getting heavy, you feel drowsy and sleepy. Close your eyes you are going to sleep. *Sleep!* If the subject should close his eyes before this, then you should make the proper alterations in the suggestions, for example: "Your eyes are closed, *sleep, deep, deep asleep!*" Or as the eyes close, say commandingly "SLEEP! DEEP ASLEEP!...You are going deeply, soundly asleep."

At this point the trance can be deepened somewhat by the methods previously described, but this is usually not done because the method you are using is designed to do this. Repeat the above procedure a number of times. Following eye closure you might give a few additional suggestions to deepen the trance, then suggestions to the effect that whenever you suggest sleep or say the word sleep, he will go quickly and deeply asleep, and will not wake up until you tell him to awaken. Then instruct him again for the next waking period. This time telling him that he will be awake and will feel fine, but that as soon as you begin to talk to him, no matter what you say, he will find that his eyes are getting heavy, difficult to keep open, that he feels tired and is getting very drowsy and sleepy and that his eyes will close and he will go into a very deep sleep, much deeper than he is now.

Somewhere along the above process you can give the subject the eye catalepsy and arm rigidity suggestions, but don't challenge him. Say something like this: "You cannot open your eyes (or you cannot bend your arm). If you tried you would be unable to do so, but you have no desire to try...Now you are relaxing...relaxing more and more, drifting down into a very deep and sound sleep." Then follow with suggestions regarding waking as previously done, or tell him that you will talk to him after he wakes up and that as soon as you mention the word "sleep," or anything that has to do with sleep, he will feel an overpowering urge to close his eyes and go to sleep.

This procedure, like many others, has variations. Many hypnotists do not bother to give suggestions, but merely dehypnotize and rehypnotize the subject repeatedly. An excellent variation of the Vogt method that often succeeds with subjects who fail to attain a deep trance is to ask them to describe the sensations they experience when going into a trance. In the next induction include suggestions describing these various feelings in the order the subject gave them to you. This feedback technique is often very effective because it prevents you from suggesting experiences the subject will not have. Some hypnotists make it a practice to ask the subject for a description of his sensations after the first induction regardless of the method used. Then on subsequent inductions the subject's own experiences are suggested as part of the induction.

MODULE 12 -- ASSESSING THE DEPTH OF HYPNOSIS

The following is an article copied from the HypnoGenesis Magazine with the permission of the author, Tom Connelly. If you are just learning hypnosis it will help you assess the depth of hypnosis your subjects have achieved.

Assessing the Depth of Hypnosis

by

Tom Connelly, BSCH, D.Hyp

After practicing hypnosis for some time we gradually develop an intuitive sense that indicates to us the depth of hypnotic trance our subjects are experiencing. This impression is probably formed inside us in a number of ways but at the beginning of our training we have to rely on a mixture of guesswork and knowledge 'borrowed' from hypnosis books, videos and our tutors.

The obvious way to make an estimate of the ongoing success of your hypnosis is to watch for the 'classic' indications of the deepening hypnotic state. Some of the following might be observed:

- *Stillness*
- *Change of breathing*
- *Pallid / waxen complexion*
- *Postural slumping*
- *REM type eye movements*
- *Eyelid fluttering*
- *Swallowing/gulping*
- *Increased Lachrymation*
- *Redness around the eyes*
- *etc.*

You will be taught to watch for these signs (and others) at the beginning of any hypnosis course of tuition but accurate assessment of trance depth only really happens when the hypnotist can evaluate these signs from personal experience. An important part of this learning process takes place when the hypnotist takes the part of the subject and experiences hypnosis from the point of view of his prospective clients. After being hypnotized many times the hypnotherapist gains an inside perspective of the mental processes that take place and an empathy for the physical nature of hypnosis. Good experience can also be had from experimenting with self-hypnosis and relaxation techniques.

Apart from personal experience of hypnosis it's possible to learn a great deal from verbal feedback. Don't be afraid to ask your subjects about their experience of trance, most will be happy to describe the 'feeling' of hypnosis and many interesting insights can be gained. Remember that hypnosis is a subjective experience and although there are many common elements to it there is much that will be unique to each individual.

It's also possible to gather direct information about the process of hypnosis and depth of trance by using a fractionation type of induction.

With the fractionation method of inducing hypnosis the process is broken into stages and the subject is questioned at each point for a verbal description of their particular experience. So the novice hypnotist can learn a great deal about the experience of relaxation and trance as it occurs in others.

The main Idea behind the fractionation method of inducing hypnosis (sometimes known as Vogt's fractionation) is to discover the personal experience of the subject as they begin to enter trance and then to 'feed back' this information to take them deeper. Subjects are relaxed into the early stages of trance and then roused and questioned for their particular experience of hypnosis and this information is then used to help the subject to go deeper still. So in a very real sense the subject is describing the best way that they personally should be hypnotized! This type of induction is not as quick as other methods but it's interactive nature does seem to lead to the deeper trance states. This method of inducing hypnosis is outlined in most good tuition courses and books but as it is outside the scope of this article the student is advised to search this information out.

Apart from methods of assessing depth of trance through observation there are also physical tests that give the hypnotist valuable information about the ongoing state of hypnosis.

The most common test is for catalepsy, usually of the eyelids. Here the subject is asked to relax the muscles of the eyelids deeply, so deeply that the eyelids will not open. This is an excellent test of relaxation, susceptibility and willingness to co-operate with the hypnosis process.

It is also possible to ask the patient to look upwards with their eyes (the head remaining still) as if at a point at the top of the head and when they have done this you can inform them that they cannot open their eyelids. It is typically quite hard to open one's eyelids with the eyes looking upwards and this might help to convince your subject of the efficacy of your techniques but it is also quite a well-known physiological 'trick' and might just as easily arouse suspicion.

Another test to gauge the level of relaxation that has the added benefit of allowing you to test for an increase in body temperature (which indicates a medium deep trance state) is the hand lift technique. After first informing your subject (who's eyes will no doubt be closed) that you are going to lift their hand, gently raise it up and let it go. The hand of a relaxed person will flop limply back. Notice how limp, warm and pliant the hand seems. Suggestions can be added to this testing technique. For example you might suggest "that as your hand falls limply down, you can go deeper and deeper into hypnosis", "as your hand falls to your lap you will go twice as deeply into relaxation."

Finally a cognitive technique to test trance depth, which does not rely on observation or physical testing. Here the hypnotist tests for amnesia (an important hypnotic phenomenon) usually by asking the subject to begin counting backwards from 300 (the actual number is not too important but it must be sufficiently large to be out of the range of 'automatic' counting) and suggesting that a point will soon be reached when the numbers will be forgotten. If a suitable trance state exists the suggestion will be accepted and the subject will forget the numeric train of thought. This method has the additional benefit that even if the subject doesn't have the correct depth of trance at that moment, the counting process may well help to bring it about!

For most practical purposes the hypnotherapist will be more concerned with establishing that there is sufficient trance depth for therapy, rather than the more academic pursuit of gauging the precise depth of trance attained. There seems to be a consensus of opinion from most learned sources that trance depth might not be such an important concern and that effective therapy can take place providing at least a light stage of hypnosis is established. This may well be the case but obtaining a medium to deep hypnotic state has two advantages:

- It inspires confidence in the hypnotist, which improves personal performance and is detected, however subliminally, by the subject.
- It is a hypnotic convincer and while it might not be any more therapeutic than a light trance state it is more of a contrast to normal waking consciousness and so helps to persuade the subject to persuade themselves that something 'significant' has taken place.

Throughout this short article I have used the convention of dividing the depth of hypnotic trance into three stages - light, medium and deep, as this seems quite sufficient for my purposes. I should point out however that there are several systems of classification, some more ancient than others. The difference

82

is usually one of division and nomenclature as the nature of the state must be a constant but the student may encounter the following descriptions depending on the source of information: i.e., Lethargy, Catalepsy and Somnambulism or Hypnoidal, Somnambulism, Coma / Esdaile state, Hypnosis attached to sleep.

It is important to realize that the 'depth of trance' does not refer to an objective or quantifiable state but is characterized by the phenomena available in that state, thereby equating trance depth with suggestibility. For example, eyelid catalepsy is quite easy to obtain and so when this phenomenon becomes available we can label the trance depth as 'light'. Pain control becomes available as a hypnotic phenomenon only when the subject becomes more suggestible and when this phenomenon becomes accessible we can label this a medium trance depth, and so on. Full amnesia or positive / negative hallucination are among the most extreme of hypnotic phenomena and require the greatest suggestibility and so when these become available we can label this a deep trance state.

In Module 13 we will return to induction techniques. We hope to cover the induction of hypnosis using imagery (picture visualization) and the Sensorimotor method (Hypnotizing without suggestions of sleep). Also, indirect methods of trance induction (inducing hypnosis without the subject's knowledge), "Drug Hypnosis," converting natural sleep into hypnosis and the Color Contrast method of inducing hypnosis.

MODULE 13 -- INDUCTION OF HYPNOSIS III

SENSORIMOTOR METHOD

(Hypnotizing Without Suggestions of Sleep)

Using this method a subject cannot only be hypnotized without reference to sleep, but without his awareness that he is being hypnotized. This method does require a lot of skill on the part of the hypnotist. The postural sway method is actually a form of the sensorimotor method of trance induction. When practicing the waking suggestions exercises, you may have found that some of your subjects passed into a condition no different than hypnosis, especially when using a series of progressively more complex waking suggestions. W.R. Wells wrote about "waking hypnosis" as the result of using waking suggestions. He began by talking to his subjects about involuntary ideomotor action and about the phenomena that happens naturally to persons in their everyday life (dissociation phenomena). He followed this with a few preliminary exercises, then asked the subjects to fix their visual attention upon some small object. He then gave the subjects suggestions of eyelid catalepsy, using the methods described in previous modules, except he did not place his finger on the subject's forehead. If this was successful, he proceeded to produce other muscular contractures (i.e., hand clasping, arm rigidity, etc.). If the eye closure suggestions failed, he recommended that one should go on to other suggestions and then come back to it. At the end of a "waking hypnosis" sessions he brought about dehypnotization by telling the subject that at a given signal he will return to his normal self. The term "sleep" or "waking" was never used.

The following is a Verbatim description by M.H. Adler and L. Secunda of a method used by them to induce a trance. They called it an indirect method because no direct suggestion of hypnotizing the subject or putting him to sleep is made. Although the authors have described the method in a therapy setting, it can be adapted to other situations.

We made use of two frequent complaints -- inability to relax and to concentrate -- as the only orientation to the hypnosis. After the preliminary case study, the procedure is introduced saying: "I shall teach you to relax and concentrate." The patient is interested in learning this procedure for it offers relief from symptoms in an objective manner. The patient is seated in a comfortable arm chair and is told to let all his muscles go limp; the head should be inclined slightly forward; the arms rest fully on the chair arms with the hands hanging limply over the edges. He is then asked to fix his glance on the thumb and forefinger of one of his hands. The physician then states: "I am going to ask you to close your eyes soon, but continue to concentrate on your thumb and forefinger. As you concentrate I shall count, and as I count you will become more and more relaxed. As you do so you will feel your thumb and forefinger draw closer and closer together. When they touch you will then know you are in a deep state of relaxation."

After this explanation, the patient is requested to close his eyes and concentrate on his thumb and forefinger. The physician repeats: "I shall start to count. As I count you will feel your thumb and forefinger draw closer and closer together as you become more and more relaxed. When your fingers touch, you will know you are in a deep state of relaxation." The count is synchronized with the patient's respirations, and continued indefinitely. At one hundred the formula is repeated. "Continue to concentrate on your thumb and forefinger. As I count you will feel your thumb and forefinger draw closer and closer together as you become more and more relaxed. When they touch you will know that you are in a deep state of relaxation." When the thumb and forefinger are in contact, the patient is told, "Now you know you are in a deep state of relaxation."

The movement of a larger muscle group is then undertaken. The physician continues: "As I count further you go into a deeper state of relaxation. As you do so, your left hand gradually, and without effort on your part, moves from the arm rest and comes to rest on the chair beside you." When this occurs, the patient is told: "Now you know you are in a deeper state of relaxation." At this point the patient is at least in light hypnosis, i.e., inability to move a limb at suggestions of heaviness and hyperesthesia to pin prick.

To bridge the gap between light hypnosis and deep trance, the suggestion of Erickson is followed. It differs only in that the words "sleep" and "trance" are omitted: "Without further counting you will continue to relax more and more, as you do so, your hand will rise without effort, and touch your face. However, your hand will not and must not touch your face until you are in the deepest state of relaxation. Then the touching of your face will be a signal that you are in a profound state of relaxation."

When this has been accomplished, a brief orientation procedure is gone through, i.e., "What is your name?" "What are you doing?" At this point the patient can be tested for depth of trance; however, deep hypnosis is not required for therapeutic results.

The patient is then trained for future induction into the same depth of trance he had attained by suggesting to him that from now on, as the physician counts from 1 to 20, he will go into this depth of relaxation and at this point his hand will rise automatically and touch his face, as a signal that he has reached the required depth of trance.

To return the patient to his non-hypnotic state the physician says: "As I count from 1 to 5, you will gradually awaken -- at 5 you will be wide awake."

After the patient awakens he usually asks whether he has been asleep or hypnotized. Whichever term he uses is then accepted by the physician who then confirms what has occurred, using the phenomena as reassurance for the patient's ability to relax under adverse circumstances. Then a discussion follows on the use of the technique to obtain subconscious and repressed material, and an opportunity is given to the patient to express his opinions on what has occurred. Since no attempts are made in the first session to produce hypnotic or posthypnotic amnesia, the patient recollects the entire process. No patient has every expressed objections to the matter in which he was introduced to hypnotherapy.

J. H. Conn described a similar technique that he used to facilitate free association. After a satisfactory transference relationship ("rapport") was established he introduced the topic of relaxation and its therapeutic effects. The patient is then requested to move to a more comfortable chair. Once seated he is asked to look up at a bright object placed several inches from his eyes and just above the horizontal line of vision. At this point, Conn emphasizes that he "*carefully defines how he expects the patient to act*" by telling him that he will *not* fall asleep so they can communicate when complete relaxation takes place. Suggestions of progressive relaxation are then given, followed by suggested eye closure. Simultaneously the bright object is gradually lowered below the line of vision. Although progressively deeper relaxation is suggested, the word sleep is never mentioned again. In some cases the eyes remained open and staring, in which case the hypnotist should ask the patient to close them. The entire procedure takes 3 to 5 minutes.

Once he obtained some overt signs of hypnosis he brings up the matter of free association by telling the subject that if anything comes to mind while he is relaxed and he feels like talking, he should do so, but that it should come without making any effort, just as easy as *breathing*. From this mention of breathing, he instructs the subject to "breathe in" and "breathe out" in a rhythmic manner. He tells the subject that this will keep him "listening" and close to the waking state. From this point on the procedure is directed at obtaining free association.

Picture Visualization

(A Semi-Indirect Method of Trance Induction)

This interesting and ingenious technique of induction was reported by M. V. Kline. He found it to be particularly effective with refractory subjects. He claims that a light to medium trance can be obtained in about 10 minutes. He referred to the procedure as a "visual imagery technique." He divides the procedure into five steps. We will now quote Kline in his own description of the method:

1. In the waking state with the eyes open, each subject was asked to visualize in "his mind's eye" certain familiar objects. In order these were: (a) a house, (b) a tree, (c) a person, and (d) an animal. The

psychodiagnostic value of this imagery production will be dealt with elsewhere. This step was continued until each stimulus had been achieved. In this population of 15 subjects, (all of whom had proven refractory to the usual techniques) all were able to achieve the requested images readily and easily. For subjects who may have difficulty in visual imagery, other methods may have to be devised based upon the principles described here.

2. Following the attainment of image formation in the waking state, each subject was told, "Close your eyes and in your mind's eye visualize yourself as you are here; sitting in the chair (or lying on the couch) *except the image of yourself has his (her) eyes open."*

3. At this point the subject was told to concentrate on the image and that all the therapist's (experimenter's) comments would be directed toward the subject's *image* and *not* toward the subject.

4. Then, a simple ocular-fixation technique was described and related to the eye-closure of the *image*. Close clinical observation of the subject will reveal subtle response patterns indicating the associative effect upon him directly. The subject can be asked to confirm eye-closure in the image, though often his straining to raise his eyebrows will reveal the situation. The image can be challenged on the lid catalepsy depending on the value that this mechanism may have in the total hypnotic relationship. Following eye-closure in the *image*, suggestions for "deepening" the trance are given in the usual manner.

5. The next step involves moving directly into the induction relationship with the *subject*. This may be done by saying, "Now you are feeling just like the image, going deeper and deeper asleep (or an equated word) and the image is disappearing." Within a few minutes, depending on the subject's personality, you will have obtained a light to medium hypnotic trance. Further depth may be secured in the usual manner, but the patient is now ready for hypnotherapeutic work.

A similar technique combined with the hand levitation method has been described by A. A. Moss. He asks the subject to select something he has seen (i.e., a movie, TV show, baseball game, etc.) and then try to recall it in exact detail and to keep it in mind. Also, the subject is told that his right arm will rise when he sees a faithful reproduction of the scene he has selected. Moss then waited for a short period. If nothing happened, he urges the subject to concentrate more, and tells him again that his hand will rise when he sees the picture. This is followed immediately with suggestions of hand levitation. As soon as the hand begins to rise, he urges the subject to keep the picture in mind and pay attention to nothing else. At this point he also adds suggestions of sleep: "...as you keep looking at the picture you are going into a pleasant deep sleep. Deeper and deeper. Sleep! Deeply! Deep sleep!" Moss then takes the subject's right arm and raises it up and forward. At the same time he tells the subject his arm will bend and his hand will move toward his face and touch it, and at that moment he will go into a deep sleep. He also suggests that the subject will continue to see the picture. He then suggests that the arm is bending, etc. When the hand touches the face, he says in a firm voice, "Deep sleep! Deep sleep!" and returns the subject's hand to his lap (if the subject does not do this himself).

Another method of hypnotization by image visualization is described by M. Powers. He has the subject, with his eyes closed, visualize a large blackboard. As soon as the subject reports he sees the blackboard, Powers tells him to visualize himself drawing a large circle on the board. Following this, he is asked to mentally draw a large "X" in the center of the circle. If he is successful, he is then asked to erase the whole picture from his mind. The subject is then again asked to visualize the empty circle and told to visualize, then erase, each letter of the alphabet in consecutive order. Powers verifies that the subject successfully enters the first few letters, then instructs him to continue, and makes no father check. As the subject continues with the letters, suggestions of deep hypnotic sleep are given. Powers claims this method is particularly effective with individuals who have a low attention span.

An Indirect Method of Trance Induction

This ingenious procedure used to induce hypnosis without the subject's knowledge, under circumstances when it is probable the subject would not have been willing to be hypnotized, was reported by E. M. Erickson and L. S. Kubie. The subject was a patient who was known to have a roommate. The roommate was contacted and her cooperation in the procedure was obtained. The patient was then requested to act as a chaperone while her roommate, who she believed to be a patient of Erickson, was being hypnotized. At the first hypnotization Erickson suggested that the patient pay close attention to the hypnotic procedure because she might someday wish to try it also. The remainder of the process is described in the author's own words:

Upon entering the office, the two girls were seated in adjacent chairs and a prolonged, tedious, and laborious series of suggestions were given to the roommate who soon developed an excellent trance, thereby setting an effective example for the intended patient. During the course of the trance, suggestions were given to the roommate in such a way that by imperceptible degrees they were accepted by the patient as applying to her. The two girls were seated not far apart in identical chairs, and in such a manner that they adopted more or less similar postures as they faced the hypnotist; also they were so placed that inconspicuously the hypnotist could observe either or both of them continuously. In this way it was possible to give a suggestion to the roommate that she inhale or exhale more deeply, so timing the suggestion as to coincide with the patient's respiratory movements. By repeating this carefully many times it was possible finally to see that any suggestion given to the roommate with regard to her respiration was automatically performed by the patient as well. Similarly, the patient having been observed placing her hand upon her thigh, the suggestion was given to the roommate that she places her hand upon her thigh and that she should feel it resting there. Such maneuvers gradually and cumulatively brought the patient into a close identification with her roommate, so that gradually anything said to the roommate applied to the patient as well.

Interspersed with this were other maneuvers. For instance, the hypnotist would turn to the patient and say casually, "I hope you are not getting too tired waiting." In subsequent suggestions to the roommate that she was tired, the patient herself would thereupon feel increasing fatigue without any realization that this was because of a suggestion that had been given to her. Gradually, it then became possible for the hypnotist to make suggestions to the roommate, while looking directly at the patient, thus creating in the patient an impulse to respond, just as anyone feels when someone looks at one, while addressing a question or comment to another person.

Once deep hypnosis was induced (which took an hour and a half) the authors took a number of measures to insure continuance of the trance, cooperation of the subject while in it, and that there would be future opportunity to use hypnotherapy. The patient was gently made aware that she was hypnotized. She was also told that nothing would be done to her that she did not want done, and there would be no need for a chaperone in the future. She was told that she could break the trance if the hypnotist should offend her. We will continue to quote the authors:

Finally, technical suggestions were given to the patient to the effect that she should allow herself to be hypnotized again, that she should go into a sound and deep trance, that if she had any resistances toward such a trance she would make the hypnotist aware of it *after* the trance had developed, whereupon she could then decide whether or not to continue in the trance. The purpose of these suggestions was merely to make certain that the patient would again allow herself to be hypnotized with full confidence that she could if she so chose disrupt the trance at any time. This illusion of self-determination made it certain that the hypnotist would be able to swing the patient into a trance. Once in that condition, he was confident that he could keep her there until his therapeutic aims had been achieved.

Although the above method is described in a therapeutic setting and involves the cooperation of a roommate, it can be adapted to other situations. It is not uncommon, as will be seen in the next module, while giving hypnotic demonstrations before groups, to find some members of the group responding to the suggestions unintentionally. This can be used to obtain additional subjects. Frequently a sudden shift of attention to these individuals with a strong command of "Sleep!" will put them into a trance.

"Drug Hypnosis"

Not a lot is known about the effects of drugs on suggestibility and hypnosis. Three things are fairly well known: 1. Narcotics of all kinds can seemingly increase waking suggestibility if given in proper dosage. 2. It is often much easier to induce hypnosis following the administration of these drugs. In some cases the drugs allow the induction of hypnosis in otherwise refractory subjects. 3. These same drugs produce other effects when given in similar dosages, such as release of emotional material, breakdown of inhibition, hyperamnesia, regression and amnesia. These effects may not be related to hypnosis, but it too can produce them. Possibly this is because, as Wolberg suggested, hypnosis and drugs partially act upon the same cortical loci. It has been shown by Brazier and Finesinger that barbiturates depress the frontal lobes first, then the motor cortex and occipital lobes.

Nowhere, as far as I know, has it ever been demonstrated that any drug by itself induces a hypnotic state. At present all we can really say is that certain drugs (i.e., any strong depressant of the nervous system) can be used as an aid in inducing hypnosis by the Standard method or related techniques. They do seem to increase waking suggestibility. However, the exact action of these drugs on suggestibility is far from clear.

Narcotics may indirectly aid in inducing hypnosis because they produce many of the symptoms of sleep that we suggest to the subject in the verbal part of the induction procedure. In the early stages of inducing hypnosis it is the temporal contiguous association of the response with the suggestion that the response is taking place or will take place that is important; not what causes the response to actually take place. If drugs will produce the suggested symptoms in the correct time frame, then we can well expect that drugs will help in the production of hypnosis.

In the early history of hypnotism, chloroform and Cannabis indica were first used as adjuncts to suggestions. When the barbiturates were developed there was a shift to there use. They proved to be safer, have a rapid action and their effect wears off quickly. Also their effects on the subject can be better graded and the optimal dosages determined. If the dose is too small the subject's suggestibility is not affected. To large a dose will depress the subject too much. We will list some of the dosages preferred by those who have had considerable experience with this technique.

Among the earlier experts, Schilder and Kauders recommended using 0.5 to 1 gm. (Maximum 1.5 gm) of Medinal. They claim quicker action can be obtained with 4 to 12 gm. But with a too rapid induction of narcosis you are more likely to miss the critical range when hypnosis can be induced, or you may not have time to produce hypnosis.

E. Stungo used Evipal sodium, about a 10 percent solution that was injected intravenously at the rate of 1 cc./min. He found that 1 to 3 cc. are required. To determine when the subject had reached the proper stage he had him count backward. When the subject began to display confusion he took this as a signal the subject had reached the desired stage. He then tried to maintain this level of sedation by continuous injection.

Wolberg recommended 6 to 9 gr. of Sodium Amytal be taken orally 30 minutes prior to hypnosis, or 1 to 2 drams of paraldehyde be taken 5 to 10 minutes before induction of the trance. If the preceding failed he suggested using intravenous injections of other drugs. He recommended 1 gm. Sodium Amytal in 30 or 40 cc. of distilled water injected at a rate of 1 to 2 cc./min.; or 7.5 gr. Sodium Pentothal in 20 cc. distilled water given in a similar manner.

Horsley in his book "Narco-analysis" states that 2 cc. of Sodium Pentothal (presumably a 2.5 percent solution) is usually sufficient, but for anxious individuals 4 cc. may be necessary. In a later book "Narcotic Hypnosis" he recommended giving orally 3 gr. of Nembutal about 30 minutes prior to the induction of hypnosis. According to him the choice of the drug used depends upon whether the patient was an in-patient or out-patient. Long-acting drugs like Nembutal are recommended with in-patients and short-acting drugs like Pentothal with outpatients.

As a rule the barbiturates used intravenously should be injected slowly with the patient counting backward. As soon as the patient becomes incoherent in counting the injection should be interrupted. This level of sedation should then be maintained. Rapport should be made prior to the injection and should be continued during and throughout the narcosis.

The standard practice using these drugs to induce hypnosis is to give a sub-anesthetic dose, just enough to cause a state of confusion and relaxation. Once the proper sedation has been obtained the subject is given suggestions aimed at inducing hypnosis proper, testing and deepening the trance as usual.

Natural Sleep and Hypnosis

Many early writers on hypnosis (and some modern ones) spoke of natural sleep being converted or passing into the hypnotic state. Some spoke of giving suggestions directly to the sleeping individual who, presumably, remained asleep. Suggestions can be effectively given to an individual who is initially asleep. However, it is debatable just what the individual's real condition is at the time the suggestions take effect. Hull has argued that when a suggestion is given to a sleeper and it is effective, he always awaken to some degree and then passes into a hypnotic state. Hull also claims that sleep is never converted directly into hypnosis, nor are suggestions ever effective if natural sleep is present. Data reported by N. Barker and S. Burwin seems to support this position.

The method consists of speaking to the sleeping person in a soft whispered monotone. Something like this is said to him: "Sleep. Remain deep asleep. You are sleeping deeply but you can hear me. You will not wake up, but you will listen to what I tell you. You are comfortable. My voice does not bother or disturb you. You are going deeper asleep, deeper all the time. But you keep hearing me. You can understand everything I tell you, but you are going more deeply asleep all the time. You will not wake up until I tell you. Remain deep asleep. You hear everything I say. You will now raise your hand to indicate to me that you can hear me. You are now raising your hand, but you will remain deep asleep." After the subject has responded to a few suggestions, tell him that even though you are going to speak louder, he will remain deep asleep. Continue to suggest sleep while raising your voice gradually until you speak in a normal tone of voice. After this proceed with whatever suggestions you want to give.

Color Contrast Method

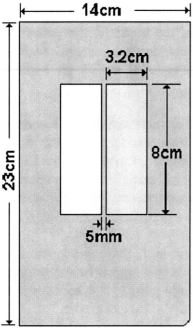

Figure 13-1

The following method was first reported by B. Stokvis. A piece of plain gray cardboard 14 by 23 cm. is used. On it two strips of paper 8 by 3.2 cm are pasted parallel to one another with a space of 5 mm. between them. The strip on the right is light blue in color and the one on the left is light yellow. Both strips have a dull finish. The lower right corner where the subject will be asked to hold the cardboard is rounded. See Figure 13-1.

The subject lying on a cough is given the cardboard and asked to hold it at arms length. He is requested to fix his gaze on the slit between the two strips. While the subject is doing this, Stokvis says:

...he is asked what he sees there. He will naturally reply "A piece of gray cardboard on which a yellow strip is pasted on the left, and a blue on the right of it, with a gray slit between." The subject is told that, as he continues to watch the picture, especially the slit, he will soon observe some additional colors appearing. These chromatic phenomena, as a general rule, will be observed physiologically by any normal person, including the so-called "red-green dichromatics," and by all "anomalous trichromatics;" they consist in appearance of the respective complementary colors along the outside edges of the yellow and blue strips.

"When you have seen the color phenomena appear, that will be proof that the hypnotic state is going to set in," I tell the subject. "In fact the appearance of the colors is the first sign of the effect of the hypnotic influence; it is a kind of fatigue phenomenon of the eyes," I assure him.

"In the same way as you have seen these color phenomena, you will observe some other signs of the approaching hypnotic state. Do keep looking at the slit; then you will soon see that the inner edge of the blue strip, that is to say, the edge bordering on the slit, becomes more intensely blue, while the rest of the blue slip will become a much duller shade. In precisely the same manner you will notice that the part of the yellow immediately bordering on the gray slit becomes more intensely yellow, while the rest of the yellow strip becomes more faintly yellow. Just keep watching sharply ... keep looking fixedly at the slit ... look very closely; you will see something else happen as well. You will also see colors appear in the slit; you will see a yellow border appear along the edge of the blue strip, and a blue border along the edge of the yellow slip. These two newly made colors will touch at about the center of the slit; now and then they will overlap; they may even disappear for a moment or two; perhaps because your consciousness is now beginning to waver, owing to the hypnotic condition, which is on the point of setting in." I will continue in this (purposely long-winded) strain.

Although the subject may perhaps feel somewhat skeptical at first toward this method of treatment, there is no doubt that by this time he will have abandoned this attitude; for he now sees before his eyes, point for point, that what is being told to him is also actually happening, with the result that his confidence in the physician will increase correspondingly.

"You remember what I told you just now" (I continue very softly and monotonously) "that, as you observe the color phenomena, you will find that your eyelids are getting heavier and heavier ... Still heavier all the time ... you will feel that you are getting more and more tired ... tired and weary ... and you will soon get so tired that you would just love to shut your eyes. When you feel like that don't resist ... don't resist ... you may close your eyes.

From this point on Stokvis' technique is the same as others. Note that he did not mention sleep anywhere in the procedure. Stokvis goes on to comment that although this technique does not usually bring about a very deep trance, there are many situations in therapy where this is not essential. Also the trance could be deepened by other means.

A method very similar to the color contrast method has been described by Powers. He recommends that the hypnotist use a pencil flashlight and aim its light into one of the subject's eyes. The subject is asked to concentrate his gaze upon the light until his eyes become heavy with fatigue. The hypnotist also tells him that he will count to five, at which time he (the subject) will close his eyes and go into a deep trance. A slow count of five is then given. If by that time the subject has not closed his eyes, he is asked to close them at his convenience. Then it is suggested that he will see a red spot inside the eye exposed to the light. He is asked to look for it and report it to the hypnotist if he sees it. When the subject reports seeing the red spot, it is suggested that it will disappear in a flash and that in its place a purple spot will appear. If the subject responds to this suggestion, other color spots are suggested. As the subject watches for color changes, suggestions of relaxation are given. From this point on the technique is one of deepening the trance.

This technique is not as subtle as Stokvis' and probably will not work with someone that has some elementary knowledge of sensory phenomena. The principle involved here is that of suggesting real sensory or perceptual effects and then suggesting very similar effects that normally would not occur. The main problem with these techniques is in preventing the subject from suspecting the true nature of his initial "hallucination."

MODULE 14 --INDUCTION OF HYPNOSIS IV

MISCELLANEOUS METHODS

Counting Methods

Seat the subject comfortably and ask him to fixate upon some object held up in front of him or have him look straight ahead at a wall. Then tell him:

I am going to begin counting and as I do I want you to follow me closely. When I say 'one' you will close your eyes and keep them closed until I say 'two.' At the count of 'two' you will open your eyes. As I say 'three' you will close them again and keep them closed until I say 'four.' Do you understand these instructions? [If the subject seems to show some confusion, demonstrate for him what you want him to do. Many hypnotists make it standard practice to demonstrate these instructions as they are given.] As I count you will continue opening and closing your eyes until they get very tired. You will find it increasingly difficult to open your eyes. They will get heavier and heavier. You will find yourself becoming more and more drowsy and sleepy. After a while your eyes will feel so heavy and you will feel so sleepy that your eyes will close and remain closed and you will go into a deep sound sleep. You will have no desire to open your eyes, you will only want to sleep, sleep deeply and soundly.

At this point begin to count in a monotonous voice, pausing after each count. Watch the subject's reactions closely. If he consistently anticipates your count, especially when opening his eyes, you may suspect he is either not paying close attention or that he is resisting. If he has difficulty opening his eyes or keeping them open, he may be entering a hypnotic state. Although it is possible to produce hypnosis by using only the counting part of the procedure, it will probably be more effective to use suggestions of heaviness of the eyelids, drowsiness, etc. These suggestions can be interjected between counts. It is a good idea to continue counting for a short time after the subject's eyes remain closed. At first, the subject may raise and lower his eyebrows in time with the count while his eyes remain close.

There are cases where a subject will continue to open and close his eyes despite becoming deeply hypnotized. This can happen if the subject does not clearly understand the instructions, or from the fact that each count acts through association as a command-suggestion. In such cases it should not be too difficult to determine if the subject is hypnotized or not. Usually he will have a fixed and blank stare if in a trance. Also his posture will assume a rigid appearance, and the motion of his eyes becomes typically automatic. Another way of determining his condition is to alter the rate of counting. If he follows these changes faithfully you can be pretty sure he is hypnotized, probably deeply. Once you have decided the subject is hypnotized, wait until he closes his eyes again, and then stop counting and say something like the following: "Now your eyes are closed and you are deep asleep. Your eyelids are very heavy...just like lead. They are stuck together...so tightly stuck together you cannot open them."

Note in the above procedure that the subject is told not to open his eyes until the next count, but is not told not to close them before the next count. This is because he may go into a deep hypnotic state and his eyes may close any time in the induction.

Metronome and Allied Methods

This method, which is closely related to the previous one, consists of having the subject listen to a metronome, a clock, watch, or a steady tone. Typically the subject is comfortably seated in a dimly lit room with his eyes closed. Having his eyes closed can be a disadvantage because there will be no way of knowing when he passes in to the hypnotic state. However, even with his eyes open, you cannot tell for sure. Because the time required for induction by this method is extremely variably, you may assume when time is at a premium that if the subject has not passed into hypnosis with in 5 to 10 minutes, he will not respond or will require much more time. For this reason, you should begin making suggestions after 5 or 10 minutes. If you have lots of time, you can allow 30 minutes to pass before starting to make suggestions. The main difficulty with this technique is that the subject may fall into a natural sleep. Often subjects who are potentially hypnotizable by this method fail to go into a trance in a short time because they do not concentrate on the sound. Sometimes it is helpful to have the subject alternately close and open his eyes with consecutive beats of the metronome.

In the classically metronome method it was assumed the subject had no knowledge of what was going to happen as he concentrated on the beats. Most hypnotists today find it more advantageous to give suggestions regarding the effects of the metronome prior to using it. Some also instruct the subjects to repeat to themselves the word "sleep" every time they hear a beat. The most effective use of the metronome seems to be in combination with suggestions. Usually an initial period of about 10 minutes is allowed without suggestions. If the subject should be responsive to the metronome alone, he will have time to manifest it.

One variation on this method consists of using a microphone to amplify the subject's heart beat or respiratory sounds. This technique makes use of two separate effects. A monotonous rhythm as a fixating stimulus. Also the rhythm of respiration acts as a conditioned stimulus for sleep. Many hypnotists believe that the metronome method works best when the rate is adjusted to some body rhythm (i.e., heart beat, respiration -- about 2 beats per second). If respiration is used, a responsive subject will adjust his rhythm to the beat of the metronome. A way to use this for the induction of hypnosis is start out with a metronome beating at a rate slightly lower than the subject's normal breathing. Ask him to breathe in unison with the metronome and pay close attention to it. This instruction should be repeated a number of times. After a few moments imperceptibly decrease the rate

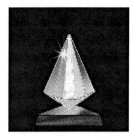

of the metronome. If the subject's breathing coincides with the metronome, change it back to the original rhythm and then increase the rhythm. If properly done, you will find that the subject adjusts his breathing to the metronome. Once this pattern has been established, suggestions of sleep can be given.

It is also possible to use a "visual metronome" (flashing light) that the subject fixates on. Actually, a combination of the two, auditory and visual stimuli can be used to an advantage.

Pendulum and Rotating Mirror Method

These are related procedures. The pendulum method makes use of a bright object attached to a chain or string. Some older hypnotists used their pocket watches which were carried at the end of a chain. The bob is held in front of the subject, slightly above eye level, and allowed to slowly swing back and forth. Suggestions as well as the beating of a metronome can be combined with this method.

The original rotating mirror method was developed by Luys. He used an old fashioned lure for meadowlarks, consisting of vertical wooden supports with many small mirrors imbedded in the surface. The device revolved about a central axis at a fairly slow rate. Subjects were instructed to concentrate on the lure. There have been many variations made of this device. One consists of one or more small glass spheres on one or more rotating arms. The subject is asked to fixate upon and follow the spheres with his eyes. As with previous techniques, suggestions can be combined with this method.

Hypnodisks and Other Devices

From the beginning of the history of hypnotism, hypnotists have tried to find some automatic and easy method of inducing hypnosis. This hope has been supported by the fact that Braid and Charcot had recourse to purely physical means to produce hypnosis. As a consequence of this search for more productive techniques, a rash of gadgets and gimmicks have been devised. Many of them have been sold (and are still being sold) as sure-fire methods of producing hypnosis. It is very doubtful any device exists that will facilitate the induction of hypnosis *in every use*. The existence of any device that induces hypnosis by a purely physical means, without the conscious participation and cooperation of the subject is very, very unlikely. It is possible that as our knowledge of hypnotism and the nervous system increases such a device may eventually be invented or discovered, but it has not been as of this time. The fact that the alpha wave can be influenced by intermittent photic and auditory stimulation and that slowing down of the alpha rhythm is symptomatic of the appearance of sleep might be used as a bases for such a device. It has been found that a flickering light can induce mental confusion, hallucinations and various other disturbed states in many people, and that in every case the disturbances were associated with specific electrical response patterns in the brain. It is conceivable that the effects of such devices as whirling spirals create similar phenomenon.

If we assume that focusing of attention is an essential factor in the induction of hypnosis, it is theoretically possible that some fixation stimuli are more effective than others, because of their greater attention-catching or compelling power. There are many such devices. For example, one device, called a hypnosphere or hypnoscope, consists of a small polished metal sphere enclosed within a larger hollow glass sphere. The presence of multiple spherical surfaces theoretically causes light placed anywhere in the room to be reflected in the subject's eyes. Also, the spherical nature of the reflecting surfaces allows the reflected lights to appear steady and relatively undisturbed by movements of the person holding the device.

Another device, called a hypnodisk or hypnotron, is a disk with a spiral (or spirals) drawn from the center. The disk is mounted on a turntable or on a shaft and rotated at a moderate speed. The subject is asked to look at the disk as he is given suggestions designed to induce hypnosis. The rational is that the apparent contracting and expanding movement gives an illusion of an axial flow which is very attention compelling. Often subjects claim that watching the disk makes them dizzy which some hypnotist capitalize on. In any event, this device appears to be one of the more effective ones. Wolberg recommends it when dealing with refractory subjects. He recommends repeating the following suggestions until the subject's eyes are closed. "Keep your eyes fastened on the wheel. As you watch it, you will notice that it vibrates. The white circles become prominent, then the black. Then it seems to recede in the distance and you feel as if you are drawn into it. Your breathing becomes deep and regular. You get drowsy, very drowsy. Soon you will be asleep."

There are several variations of the disk. One has a number of concentric rings drawn on it. The subject is requested to fixate upon it as the hypnotist rotates it. It results in an illusion that the concentric rings are turning. Another variation consists of a background of spirals covered by a piece of plastic molded so that its surface consists of a large number of tiny parallel semi cylindrical lenses. Any slight movement of the disk causes the spirals to shimmer and change.

Another method often found in book for beginners is the "candle method." The subject is required to watch the flame of a candle. Probably it effectiveness is due to the mysterious and dramatic effect of the ever changing shape of the flame. It is said that dancing flames exert a peculiar fascination on people.

It is doubtful that any of these devices are superior in speed, depth of hypnosis, or the percentage of subjects successfully hypnotized. They are also bulky to carry around. However, a professional hypnotist should avail himself of such devices because when other methods fail one of these devices may succeed.

Hypnosis by Passes

Passes are movements of the hands made by the hypnotist over the subject's body. The hands may or may not touch the body. They were originally introduced by the mesmerists on the assumption that the motions directed, concentrated or dispersed the animal magnetism upon and within the subject. Today they are used almost entirely for theatrical effect. However, if a subject believes in their effectiveness, there is a certain value in using them. According to the mesmerists passes are very important and must be used correctly or not at all. This involves special ways of holding the hands and fingers, certain mental attitudes, certain ways of moving the hands etc. There are six major types of passes:

1. *Longitudinal passes* are made head to foot with the hands a few inches from the surface of the body. Their objective is to dissipate the magnetic fluid throughout the body. They are extensively used to induce "magnetic sleep."

2. *Passes "a grand courant."* These are similar to the above but made more rapidly, with wider motions and at a greater distance from the body. They are said to have a greater effect on the subject than the longitudinal passes.

3. *Oblique passes* are a variation of (2). They differ in that the two arms describe arcs of circles in front of the subject. The object is to remove or dissipate whatever animal magnetism is present in the chest and head. They are used to awaken the subject from induced magnetic somnambulism.

4. *Transverse passes.* The arms are crossed in front of the hypnotist's chest, the palms forward facing the subject. Then the arms are rapidly stretched forward and outward. These passes are supposedly the most radical method of dissipating any magnetism accumulated at any point in the subject's body. The mesmerists consider these passes an excellent way to awaken the subject.

5. *Vibratory passes* are supposed to be the magnetizer's most powerful pass in regard to his emission of animal magnetism. They are made in a variety of ways. Different parts of the hand come into contact with the subject, with the hands stationary in one position or moving in one of the ways described above. At the same time the hands are given a continuous vibratory motion.

6. *Circular passes* are made with short or large circular motions of the hands and arms and have different qualities depending upon whether done clockwise or counterclockwise.

There is no evidence to indicate that passes have any special properties. Whether one uses them is a matter of personal choice, belief, and showmanship. Judging by past records they can be very effective.

Hyperventtilation

Voluntary hyperventilation (forced deep breathing *without forced expiration*) appears to raise a subject's suggestibility. Many hypnotists do use it to facilitate the induction of hypnosis. However, to be effective it must be maintained over a period of time and not limited to a few deep breaths. There are a number of ways of proceeding. The induction of hypnosis can be preceded by two to four minutes of hyperventilation and then followed by suggestions. Another good method is to have the subject concentrate on his breathing and take rhythmic breaths as deeply as possible in regular, rapid succession. Probably the hypnotist should set the pace at first by indicating the rhythm with movements of his hands or by saying in a monotonous voice, "in -- out," or "breathe in -- breathe out." This not only sets the pace, but getting the subject to voluntarily respond to the words of the hypnotist adds to his suggestibility. After a rhythm has been established, standard suggestions can be integrated with the breathing.

If hyperventilation is carried out to long unconsciousness can occur. This is not particularly dangerous because when the subject loses consciousness he automatically stops hyperventilating and will regain consciousness. However, this would certainly interfere with attempts at hypnotization. Normally, you

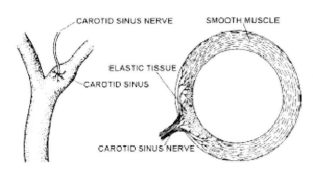

may expect subjects to enter a state of hypnosis before hyperventilation causes them to lose consciousness, however, some people are particularly susceptible to the effects of hyperventilation and may faint before hypnosis has been induced. It is actually an easy matter to check on the subject's state of awareness and the suggestibility of the subject and discontinue hyperventilation with the onset of hypnosis.

What do you do if a subject should faint? Nothing, he will shortly recover alone because fainting automatically brings an end to hyperventilation. Besides fainting, a number of other effects may be observed during hyperventilation; Sweating, cold, clammy skin, more rapid heart beat, muscular weakness and fatigue. These are normal reactions and you should not be concerned about them. However, the subject may be concerned and you may have to assure him that they are normal reactions.

The Carotid Sinus Method

High in the neck each of the major arteries (carotids) supplying blood to the brain divides into two smaller arteries. At this bifurcation, the wall of the artery is thinner than usual and contains a large number of branching, vine like nerve endings. This small portion of the artery is called the *carotid sinus*. These nerve endings are highly sensitive to stretch and distortion. Applying pressure to them can trigger a syndrome that affects the flow of blood, oxygen and carbon dioxide in the blood, heart rate, blood pressure and other functions.

One of the main attractions of the carotid sinus method is it great speed of action, its *apparent* simplicity and the *false* assumption that it is a sure fire technique requiring little skill on the part of the hypnotist. The carotid sinus technique is based on a known physiologic phenomenon that often results in a state of unconsciousness when carried to completion. THIS IS A DANGEROUS PROCEDURE THAT HAS NO PLACE IN THE REPERTOIRE OF THE HYPNOTIST. This procedure triggers an entire syndrome, which among other things can cause the heart to stop. There are numerous records of instantaneous deaths caused through the elicitation of the carotid sinus reflexes. Also it is difficult to use these reflexes to produce hypnosis because their action is often to rapid, variable, and difficult to

97

control. It is doubtful, even when used by an expert, that it has anything but "show" value. One thing is certain; the collapse of the subject following the elicitation of the syndrome is not hypnosis, although some less than honest stage hypnotists have often indicated otherwise.

The actual production of hypnosis using this technique involves giving the subject proper suggestions while he is passing from consciousness to unconsciousness. With many subjects this in-between state can be fairly easily maintained. With others it is extremely brief in time.

Rapid Methods

In modern times stage hypnotists have placed much emphasis upon "rapid hypnosis" and particularly "instantaneous hypnosis." An example of the instantaneous method is the triggering of the hypnotic state by the use of a posthypnotic signal. This will produce hypnosis in a fraction of a second. Many of the other so-called "instantaneous" methods are better described as rapid techniques that require at best a minute or more. In many cases the claims of rapid hypnosis are deceptive because they neglect to take into account the time used to prepare the subject or to "set the stage." With the exception of hypnosis produced by a posthypnotic signal, the best you can say for the rapid methods is that they very fast, *when they work*. When they fail, you are probably worse off than if you had tried a slower technique in the first place. However, there is no question that under the proper conditions rapid hypnosis is possible.

If a person has a high suggestibility quotient, and feels you are a "powerful" hypnotist, a sudden look from you with a firm command of "sleep!" will sometimes be sufficient to induce a state of hypnosis. This is particularly successful if he has just witnessed the induction of hypnosis in others at a signal or command by you.

Sometimes when a subject appears a little dazed, eyes glazed, and unstable on his feet after responding well to a few waking suggestions will go into a hypnotic state if you suddenly look at him and command, "sleep." This is especially true after a good response to the postural sway experiment. A simple but effective technique is to quickly extend your hand toward the subject's face; snap your fingers near his eyes and at the same time command "*Sleep! Deep asleep!*" If done properly, the eyelids will close due to a reflex if not as the result of hypnosis and will remain closed if the subject is sufficiently suggestible. Another technique is to watch nearby people in an audience while giving a demonstration of hypnosis. It is not uncommon to find someone in the audience showing evidence of being influenced by the proceedings. Very often if you turn toward him and command sleep, he will be deeply hypnotized.

One very effective method used by many stage hypnotists is to start giving the postural sway suggestions and as the subject begins to fall, step back so that their chest will support the head and shoulders of the subject when he is caught. As he comes to rest against the hypnotist's chest the hypnotist slides one hand over the subject's eyes, forcing him to close them. At the same time the command "*Sleep! Deep, deep sleep!*" is given. Then suggestions to deepen the trance are given before the subject is helped back to a normal standing position.

Even the Chevreul pendulum demonstration can be used to induce hypnosis. The subject is asked to concentrate on the bob and its motion. When movement is obtained, he is told he cannot stop it and is

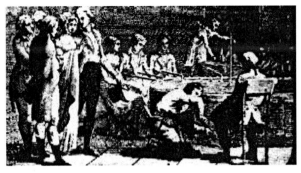

challenged to do so. Depending on his reaction, you can command sleep or begin a slower induction of hypnosis. With a subject that fails to meet the challenge, a trance can often be induced by stating in a positive manner "All right, now you can stop it if you wish, but you are getting very sleepy. *Sleep!* DEEP ASLEEP!" This command can be emphasized by snapping your fingers next to his eyes.

The problem with all of these methods is that they are very uncertain. Their success depends too much on the hypnotist's ability to pick the proper subjects and to adequately set the stage. The ability to detect if a subject is ready for these techniques is somewhat of an art. A tense, fixed expression, bodily tenseness, expectancy and glazed eyes are among the cues an experienced hypnotist looks for.

These methods are rarely recommended for the beginner's use. The only true method of instantaneous hypnosis is the use of a posthypnotic signal. While the subject is hypnotized you suggest to him that the next time you give a particular signal he will immediately go into a deep sleep. Any signal will do. It is a good idea to suggest that he will not recall this. While this is a simple and effective technique, it is not foolproof. Of course, the subject has to be hypnotized the first time before it can be used. Although posthypnotic suggestions can be effective with a light trance, to be fully effective and lasting, the subject should be in a deep hypnotic state, or at least in moderately deep hypnosis. When using this technique, *you should be very careful to not use a word as a signal that you would use in an ordinary conversation with the subject.* If you do not observe this rule, you may find your subject falling into a trance when it is not intended. Also it should be made clear that he will only respond to the signal if it is given by an authorized person. Never say, "Anytime you hear the word 'rosebud' you will go into a trance," or even "Anytime someone says 'rosebud' to you."

MODULE 15 - INDUCTION OF HYPNOSIS V

CLASSICAL METHODS

Mesmerism -- The Magnetic Method

Franz Anton Mesmer

Around the time of the American Revolution, Franz Anton Mesmer   (1733   - 1815), a Viennese physician, introduced to the scientific world the theory and practice of what he called animal magnetism. The spirit of the times tinged his practice with something of the mystical. In 1778 he went to Paris where he opened a clinic that became tremendously successful. In his remarkable clinic he treated all kinds of diseases.

Copy of old drawing of Mesmer's Baque

His clinic consisted of a large hall, which was darkened by covering the windows. In the center of the room was a large oaken tub, the famous *baquet*. The tub, about one foot high, was big enough to allow thirty patients to stand around it. The tub was filled with water, in which had been placed iron filings, ground glass and several bottles arranged in a symmetrical manner. The tub had a wooden cover that contained openings through which jointed iron rods protruded. The patients could apply these rods to the various ailing parts of their bodies. At a strategic moment, Mesmer would appear dressed in brilliant silk robes. He would pass among the patients, fixing his eyes upon them, passing his hands over their bodies, and touching them with a long iron wand. Patients apparently suffering from various disorders would declare themselves cured after two to three treatments.

Mesmerism, like psychoanalysis, embodies a theory, a set of phenomena, and a type of therapy. Hypnotism comprises a group of phenomena that can include the phenomena of mesmerism, however, it is questionable whether all the results reported by Mesmer and his students are true manifestations of hypnosis. For example, according to Mesmer, a successful treatment by animal magnetism ended in what he called the "crisis" which was a convulsive attack usually accompanied by crying and laughing. His "crisis" had all the earmarks of hysteria, which may have played a part in some of the results.

The essence of mesmerism can be found in his doctoral dissertation (1766) in which he theorized upon the influence of emanations from heavenly bodies on the health of human beings. Shortly after writing this he became aware of the work of a priest who was said to obtain miraculous results in the art of healing by exposing his patients to the influence of magnets. Mesmer came to believe that magnets emanated two sources of influence: physical magnetism, which he called "mineral magnetism" and the other, which had analogous properties, he called "animal magnetism." He identified animal magnetism as the universal emanation he had hypostatized in his dissertation. According to Mesmer, animal magnetism had the following properties: it could be transferred to animate and inanimate bodies; it could become concentrated or diffused by such bodies; it could act at a distance; it could be reflected by mirrors; it could be communicated, propagated, and increased by sound; it could be accumulated in bodies; and it had two polarities which could produce opposite effects and could decrease or destroy each other's effects. It was thought to be a kind of impalpable gas or fluid. Its distribution and action were supposed to be under the control of the human will.

Mesmer's sole interest in animal magnetism was due to its curative powers. According to him, a patient's health depended upon the distribution of animal magnetism in his body. Ill health was do to an excess or a deficiency of animal magnetism in the patient's entire body, or in specific parts of his body. Mesmer cured patients of their maladies by giving, removing or redistributing the animal magnetism within the patient.

Later magnetizers developed these ideas into a somewhat impressive body of pseudo-scientific knowledge. In time negative or positive animal magnetism became associated with every known physical phenomenon and object. Also, it became capable of acting as a medium of transmission for various properties of the objects from which it came. For example, various effects of drugs were said to be transported at a distance by their animal magnetism. Also, human thought and the will could be affected and carried by it. Certain individuals, called "sensitives," were said to be able to see animal magnetism. It appeared to them as a luminous emanation, or "aura" surrounding all individuals and objects. It was claimed that this "aura" varied in color and intensity for each individual and changed as his thoughts and emotions changed. As this doctrine was embellished, it was used to account for various reported supernormal phenomena. For example, phantasms or "astral projections" were said to be nothing but exteriorized animal magnetism or that which had become released from its owner's body upon death. It was also believed that animal magnetism could be used as a medium for communication via thoughts.

One of the most spectacular applications of this doctrine was made by de Rochas, a follower of the Salpetriere school. He claimed to have proof that under hypnosis one could extract or project the subject's sensory capacities with his animal magnetism and impregnate objects with the latter, transferring these capacities to the object. He claimed, anything done to the object was felt by the subject, no matter how far apart they were.

The above is a very brief and incomplete account of the doctrine of animal magnetism and its ramifications. It is an extremely fascinating subject if for no other reason than it represents one of the most complete misrepresentations of facts under the guise of science. It demonstrates how suggestibility and the desire to believe can lead to a fantastic adulteration of information.

BRAIDISM -- The Beginnings of Modern Hypnosis

In 1841, James Braid an English physician witnessed a mermeric seance conducted by a French magnetizer named Lafontaine. He attended the demonstration expecting fraud. Upon seeing the demonstration a second time and making certain tests on the magnetized subjects himself, he became convinced that the phenomena were real. He became enthusiastic about what he saw and experimented on his own. His experiments soon lead him to believe that the cause of the various phenomena was *not* a fluid that passed from the body of the mermerist into the subjects.

Braid developed a special technique for inducing the trance, a method still used to this day. He originally had his patients look at a cork attached to his forehead. He later replaced the cork with a bright object held near and slightly above the eyes in such a way that the eye muscles were under a certain amount of strain. The subjects were instructed to look fixedly at the object. This procedure was usually combined with verbal suggestions. It was braid that coined the word *hypnotism*. He utilized the trance mainly for painless surgical operations of which he performed in large numbers.

The following is Braid's own account of his procedure for inducing the hypnotic trance:

Take any bright object (I generally use my lancet case) between the thumb and forefinger and middle fingers of the left hand; hold it from about eight to fifteen inches from the eyes, at such position above the forehead as may be necessary to produce the greatest strain upon the eyes and eyelids, and enable the patient to maintain a steady fixed stare on the object. The patient must be made to understand that he is to keep his eyes steadily fixed on the object, and the mind riveted on the idea of the object. It will be observed, that owing to the consensual adjustment of the eyes, the pupils will be at first contracted; they will shortly begin to dilate, and after they have done so to a considerable extent, and have assumed a wavy motion, if the fore and middle fingers of the right hand, extended and a little separated, are carried from the object toward the eyes, most probably the eyelids will close involuntarily, with a vibratory motion. If this is not the case, or the patient allows the *eyeballs* to *move*, desire him to begin anew, giving him to understand that he is to allow the eyelids to close when the fingers are again carried toward the eyes, but that the *eyeballs must be kept fixed in the same position*, and the *mind riveted to the one idea of the object held above his eyes.* It will generally be found that the eyelids close with a *vibratory* motion, or become spasmodically closed.

He states that after the hypnotic state is obtained, you can place the limbs of the subject in any position and they will remain that way. After a while he claimed, the limbs tend to become rigid and involuntarily fixed. He also claimed that all of the sense organs (except sight), muscular motion, resistance and certain mental faculties *first* become extremely *elevated*. Later there appears a very large *depression* in the form of a profound *torpor* accompanied with tonic rigidity of the muscles.

The scientific formulation of hypnosis began with Braid. It was due to his accurate descriptions of empirical facts. Of the three leading investigators of Mesmerism, Elliotson, Esdaile and Braid, it is Braid that made the most significant contributions. Esdaile and Elliotson were "fluidists" and radical proponents of mesmerism. Unlike the mesmerists, Braid maintained that his method of induction would not affect anyone without his or her full participation (free will). This was directly opposite the claims made by the mesmerists that they had the power to overcome a subject's resistance merely by exerting their "will power" and by secret "passes."

Braids technique was that of the modern day hypnotherapist. His approach was patient-centered, including the principle that the patient could hypnotize himself independent of the influence of another. He was opposed to the idea that hypnosis could be induced by magnets or any other type of physical device and insisted that hypnotic phenomena were subjective and induced by direct and indirect suggestion. He believed that *rapport* was an artifact created by the operator's attitude and recognized the importance of verbal and non-verbal suggestion in the development of the induction phase.

Charcot and Hypnotism

J. M. Charcot

Charcot, a famous French neurologist and anatomist, played a very important, but very controversial part in the history of scientific hypnotism. Around 1880 he attracted a lot of attention by his courageous experiments and lectures on the subject of hypnosis. Aware of the unscientific extravagances that brought the magnetizers into disrepute, he resolved that his experiments would be ultra-scientific and technically above reproach. Despite Charcot's scientific intentions, no one has ever created more errors or gone more widely afield in his experimental methods than he. The results of his research culminated in the delivery in 1882 of his famous nosographic paper before the Paris Academy of Science.

Apparently he never hypnotized anyone himself, but depended upon his assistants, who brought the subjects to him. The subjects were mainly three hysterical young women. He sought diligently to document the objective signs that characterized hypnotic sleep. He reported a number of supposed discoveries. Major hypnotism, as it was then called, was said to show three sharply marked stages: lethargy, catalepsy and somnambulism. In the lethargic stage, which was induced by closing the subject's eyes, he maintained that the subject could hear nothing and could not speak. However, if certain nerves were pressed, amazing and uniform contractures resulted. While in the lethargic stage, the cataleptic stage could be induced by opening the subject's eyes. In this state the subject's limbs remained in any position they were placed. Finally, if friction were applied to the top of the head, the subject passed into the somnambulistic stage. Sometimes the contractures, catalepsies, and other hypnotic manifestations appeared on only one side of the body. In such cases, if a strong magnet were brought close to the affected side, the symptoms would be transferred to the other side of the body.

The main problem with Charcot's nosography was that it did not agree with the observations of many of his contemporaries. Bernheim, the principal voice of the opposition, insisted that he had never witnessed the spontaneous occurrence of Charcot's syndromes. Even more damaging was his contention that only by suggesting the various symptoms could they be obtained. Bernheim's final conclusion was that the pre-education of the subjects or unwitting suggestions to them, accounted for the three stages reported by Charcot. This resulted in the now famous and often violent controversy between the Salpetriere and Nancy schools of hypnotism.

The above very brief history of hypnotism is largely only of historic and academic interest today. Like all sciences, hypnotism has descended from magic and superstition, but none has been so slow as hypnosis in shaking off the evil associations of its origin.

MODULE 16 - INDUCTION OF HYPNOSIS VI

MASS OR GROUP HYPNOSIS

Hypnotizing a large number of people at the same time is not difficult. The group can either be a selected group or an unselected group. In the first case, the subjects can be individuals that have submitted to a few tests of suggestibility (i.e., postural sway, hand clasping, etc.) and proven to be potentially good hypnotic subjects or they can be untested volunteers. As a rule, you will find that volunteers are more susceptible to hypnosis than are non-volunteers. In the second case, the entire audience is used, no testing or calling for volunteers is done.

In the case of the group selected on the bases of suggestibility tests, you can proceed in one of two ways. You can pick out a few subjects that you consider highly suggestible and hypnotize them individually before the rest of the group. Often you will find that other members of the group will also have gone to "sleep" or have become partially hypnotized. If this is the case, you can turn to them and finish hypnotizing them or deepen the trance. Tell each subject, including the ones you worked with individually: "You will remain as you are, deep asleep, until I tell you otherwise. You will not awaken until I tell you to." It is good practice to lightly touch each subject on the shoulder or arm as you address him. This will make your suggestions more emphatic and personal. Whether or not other members of the group go into a trance after you have hypnotized a few subjects individually, turn to them and say something like this: "Hypnotizing is a easy as that. Now, I want all of you to look at my eyes."

The other mode of proceeding is to hypnotize the group with out any individual demonstrations. You can start with a group of volunteers or the entire audience by demonstrating waking suggestions or even hypnosis with a few subjects picked from the group. Alternately, you can give the entire audience waking suggestions as explained in module 9. Most hypnotists will only give the hand-clasping test to the entire audience. Then ask those that had difficulty, or are unable to separate their hands, to come forward and act as subjects. If you are dealing with a group of volunteers, you can very effectively turn the hand-clasping test into a trance-inducing procedure. When the test is concluded you can go directly into suggestions of sleep.

Once you have exhausted the volunteers and the subjects selected by means of a test, you probably have not gotten all the good subjects in the audience. Some of the best subjects may still be in the audience. For this reason, when you are ready to hypnotize the selected group, tell the audience something like this: "Shortly I am going to ask those who have volunteered to perform an exercise in relaxation. You may try it also if you wish. I think you will find it very interesting. All you have to do is close your eyes and listen to what I tell you and do what I tell you. Now just close your eyes." Then turn to the volunteer group and say: "Those of you have volunteered look into my eyes."

Alternately, you can address the volunteers first and give them some preliminary instructions. Say to them: "In a moment we will do an exercise in relaxation. I think you will find it very interesting. All you need to do is look at my eyes and listen to what I tell you and do what I ask you to do. Now just close your eyes." At this point turn to the audience and add: "Those of you that are watching may like to try this also. You will find it a very pleasant and interesting experience. Just close your eyes and listen to what I say. Don't worry, you will not miss anything. All right now, close your eyes and just listen." Now, turn to the subjects and proceed to induce hypnosis.

When you have finished the induction, add the following instructions: "Some of you in the audience are now sound asleep. You will remain sleeping and will not wake up until I tell you to do so. In a few moments I will have someone next to you bring you to me. You will remain deeply asleep and follow him to me. The rest of you in the audience may now open your eyes. Please look around you, if you see anyone sleeping, please bring him to me. Just take hold of his arm and help him gently out of the chair and guide him to me." You should always make it a point to come forward to meet the subject.

Other than outlined above, the induction of hypnosis in a group is virtually the same as inducing hypnosis in single individuals. One method that can be used with hardly any alterations is the first method described in module 10 (A Simple Induction).

We will now give a few samples of mass hypnosis. The following instructions assume that the audience is being address. Except for the last part of the following, the instructions are equally applicable to groups of volunteers assembled on a stage or anywhere in the room. When dealing with volunteers, there may be occasions when they are not all seated. If possible try to have as many chairs as you estimate you will have volunteers. However, *never turn down volunteers for a lack of chairs*. There is no reason why some subject cannot be kept standing. You can arrange the extra subjects in rows behind or in line with the chairs. You can then start giving your suggestions, making a few appropriate changes where needed. For example, you might say something like this: "...Those of you who are standing relax as much as possible, but hold yourself straight, hands by your sides." When the time comes to instruct the subjects to clasp their hands, specify that the standing subjects keep their clasped hands in front of them, and the sitting subjects hold them in their laps.

After making some introductory remarks to the audience, say something like the following:

I would now like to invite you to participate in an interesting experiment. Please place both of your feet flat on the floor. If you have any rings on your fingers, please remove them and place then in your pocket or handbag. Now clasp your hands together as I am doing and keep them in your lap. Breath deeply, just as I am doing. Continue breathing deeply and only listen to my voice. As you continue breathing deeply imagine that every muscle in your body is relaxing, just turn them lose, just like a hand full of loose rubber bands.

Allow a wonderful feeling of relaxation to flow into every muscle of your body. Feel your entire body relaxing. Your entire body is relaxing more and more with each easy breath you take. Now let your eyelids close and continue breathing deeply and easily. You arms and hands are beginning to feel heavy, your legs are growing heavy. Your entire body is growing heavy, heavier and heavier. You are becoming pleasantly drowsy, sleepy...

Just listen to my voice. Think of nothing but what I tell you. As you continue to relax more and more and become more and more sleepy you will find that your hands are becoming stuck together. In a few moments you will find that your hands are so tightly stuck together that you will not be able to take them apart until I tell you that you can. But for now just continue listing to my voice. Your hands are heavy, very heavy.

Your arms are heavy, very heavy. Your legs and feet are very heavy. Your entire body is very heavy, so very heavy. You are drowsy, so very drowsy, so sleepy. Just allow yourself to drift into a deep pleasant sleep. Feel yourself drifting down into a very pleasant, restful sleep. You can hear everything I say and will continue to listen to me. Nothing will disturb you. You are only aware of my voice. You feel comfortable and are going into a deep sleep. Now as I continue to speak to you, you will find that your hands are stuck together.

They are so completely stuck together that you cannot separate them. The more you try, the more tightly they stick together. You will remain asleep with your eyelids closed and as I count your hands will become more tightly stuck together. One...They are sticking tighter together. Two...they are stuck tight. Three...tighter. Four...tighter and tighter. Five...They are stuck tight, you cannot take them apart, the more you try, the tighter they stick together...

Now stop trying and relax. Now you can take your hands apart, but now your eyelids are sticking together, sticking more and more tightly closed. No matter how hard you try, you cannot open your eyes, they are stuck closed...All right now, stop trying and relax. You are going deep asleep, deep asleep. Drifting down deeper and deeper asleep.

You might then suggest that they raise their right arms above their heads and make a tight fist. Follow this with suggestions that their arms are stiff and they cannot bend them until you tell them they can. This has the triple purpose of testing suggestibility, deepening the trance and allowing you to get an idea of whom in the audience has responded to your suggestions.

At this point, you can do one of three things. Have members of the audience guide these subjects to you as described before. If practical, go to each subject and give him a few additional suggestions to deepen his trance and escort him to the place where you will give the rest of the demonstration. Or, you can instruct the subjects that they will in the future become instantaneously hypnotized when you command them to sleep; wake them up and ask them to come forward as subjects. You can then quickly hypnotize them as a group or individually.

An effective variation of this procedure is as follows. Either the entire audience or a group of volunteers are instructed to clasp their hands. Have them look at some fixation object or your eyes. If feasible, have the lights dimmed. Now ask them to breathe deeply and rhythmically. Then tell them you are going to count and as you do, they should pay close attention to the counts and what you say. Tell them not to think about anything but what you tell them. Then count something like this:

One...As I count you will feel yourself relaxing and soon you will fall asleep.

Two...You will find this an interesting and very pleasant experience.

Three...As you continue to relax more and more; a feeling of heaviness will come over you.

Four...You feel yourself getting drowsy, so sleepy.

Five...As you continue to relax and feel more and more sleepy; your hands are becoming stuck together.

Six...You hands are sticking tighter together.

Seven...Tighter.

Eight...Tighter and Tighter.

Nine...Your hands are stuck together, you cannot separate them, try!

Ten...Stop trying and go deeper asleep.

Eleven...If your eyelids are not closed, please close them.

Twelve...Let yourself go deeper and deeper asleep.

Thirteen...You are deep asleep.

Fourteen...I may awaken some of you shortly; if I do, you will go right back to sleep as soon as I tell you to.

Fifteen...Sleep deeply...Soundly. You will not awaken until I tell you. Just stay as you are until I speak to you again.

At this time, as explained before, instruct the nonhypnotized members of the audience regarding those that have entered a trance. Then, as soon as feasible, dismiss the subjects that are obviously not hypnotized. Watch for subjects that are lightly hypnotized and may tend to awaken. If you observe a subject awakening, you can usually re-induce the trance by giving him a few suggestions of sleep. It is good practice to give individual attention to each subject that is hypnotized by touching him on the shoulder or the arm. As you do you should deepen his trance and restate that he will not awaken until you tell him to. Also tell him that if he should awaken for any other reason, he will immediately go

106

back to sleep at your command. As a rule, this method will quickly hypnotize a large group of people. However, with the exception of a few, most of the subjects will be in a light to medium state of hypnosis.

A good way to deepen the trance would be to apply a variation of the fractionation method (see Module 9) by awaking the subjects, all at once or only a few at a time, under some pretext, and then re-hypnotizing them. You do not have to have all the subjects participate at the same time. However, it is a good idea to suggest to those remaining inactive, that their trance will deepen while they wait and that they will not pay any attention to what you say until you address them or give them some signal such as touching them on the shoulder. In general, you will get the best results with mass hypnosis by working quickly but smoothly and keeping your subjects performing most of the time.

The fractionation method can be used very effectively when performing group hypnosis. Tell the subjects that appear sufficiently hypnotized that you are going to awaken them and have them return to their chairs, but once they are seated, they will feel sleepy. Also tell them that as they watch you, they will get sleeper as time passes, their eyelids will get progressively heaver, so heavy that they will close and they will drift deeply asleep; and not awaken until you tell them to. Then awaken them, and have them return to their chairs.

While working with those subjects who went into satisfactory trances, keep an eye on those given the above suggestions. Often after a short time you will notice one of these subjects nodding or showing difficulty keeping his eyes open. When this occurs, point your finger at him in a rapid, sudden motion, and say in a commanding voice, "SLEEP!" This will often put him into a deep trance. In many cases these subjects will become hypnotized with out this step and you can attend to them later.

Mass hypnosis is useful when giving demonstrations and increasing the susceptibility of prospective subjects or patients. It can act as a form of psychotherapy. Mass suggestion is probably at the bottom of mass cures that have been reported to occur in temples, churches, and holy sites since ancient times. Mesmer was one of the first physicians to make use of these techniques on a large scale. Bernheim used the technique to increase the susceptibility of his patients.

MODULE 17 - ANIMAL HYPNOSIS

IMMOBILIZATION

There are four principal ways that a state of hypnosis can be induced in an animal. The methods are:

Repetitive Stimuli -- This includes scratching or stroking various areas of the body, staring into the eyes of the animal, closing the eyes of the animal and swinging it back and fourth, and suddenly presenting a very bright stimulus.

Inversion -- In many instances a sudden inversion of an animal will induce a state of hypnosis.

Pressure on Body Parts -- Often pressure applied to the abdominal region of an inverted animal will produce a state of hypnosis. This region will vary with different animals.

Restraint of Movement -- This seems to be an essential element in the production of hypnosis in animals. It is probably virtually impossible to use any of the other methods without some form of restraint of motion.

There appears to be no way of knowing which method will work best with any given animal. Some animals may not respond twice to the same method. Other my respond well to several of the methods.

The state of hypnosis in animals is manifested by a state of immobilization characterized by a condition of hypertonicity, usually associated with marked plasticity. However, relaxation and rigidity have also been observed. The state of immobility may last for several hours. During this time the animal appears to be insensitive to most stimuli. Some animals tend to go into this state more quickly and remain in this condition longer with successive repetitions of the induction process.

Because of the nature of Pavlov's study of Conditioned Reflexes he encounter the phenomenon of animal hypnosis quite often. His dogs were restrained during his experiments and subjected to monotonous situations. After extensively studying animal hypnosis he came to the conclusion that it was do to a self-protecting reflex of an inhibitory nature. Faced with an overwhelming power from which there was no escape an animal's only chance of survival is to remain immobile in order not to be noticed. The condition of immobility is triggered in the following way. The animal is subjected to external highly intense stimuli or to unusual stimuli that are capable of triggering a rapid inhibitory reflex in the motor region of the cerebral cortex that controls voluntary movements. Depending on the duration or intensity of the stimuli, this inhibition is either confined to the motor region, or it irradiates to other regions of the cerebral hemispheres all the way to the mid-brain. If it is confined to just the motor region reflexes of the eye muscles are present (i.e. the animal follows the experimenter with its eyes), and tonic reflexes from the mid-brain to the skeletal muscles cause the animal to retain the position it is placed in (catalepsy). In the second case the above-mentioned reflexes gradually disappear as the animal becomes absolutely passive with a general relaxation of the musculature. Pavlov believed this inhibition is nothing more than sleep, but partial and localized.

There has been a lot of research done in the area of animal hypnosis, however little is known about the phenomenon and there is very little agreement among investigators regarding the known facts. The methods of induction are extremely variable in there effectiveness. Very little can be done with animals in these states. There are no known applications that can be applied to human management from the studies of animal hypnosis. It is a topic of great scientific interest and in time may be of considerable value for the practical use of hypnosis.

Closed Door Self Hypnosis

Published by Velocity Group Publishing

PO Box 9516 Hamilton, NJ 08650   www.advancedmindpower.com   www.mindforcesecrets.com

Self Hypnosis
OVERVIEW

The key to learning self-hypnosis is the SEMANTIC RELAXATION EXERCISE. This exercise should take about ten to fifteen minutes. A few people who practice this exercise will develop the hypnotic state the first time they try it. The most resistant individuals will have entered the hypnotic state after practicing the exercise daily for about six weeks. Most people lie some where between the two extremes. Using this method of eliciting the hypnotic state does not require you to believe, have faith, or confidence that it will work for you. All you need to do is practice the exercise at least once a day for ten to fifteen minutes. If you would like to know why this exercise works, perform the experiment outlined in IDEOMOTOR ACTION listed on the home page under HYPNOSIS. I think you will find this experiment very interesting.

When you practice the Semantic-Relaxation exercise you should start by visualizing the muscles in the toes relaxing. Some people find it helpful to visualize the muscles as a bunch of loose rubber bands, ever becoming more and more limp and loose. Then visualize the muscles in the ball of the foot relaxing. Let yourself see them completely limp and relaxed in your imagination. Then move on to the arch of the foot. See those muscles relaxing. Then let the relaxation move into the ankles. From the ankles, let the relaxation flow into the long muscles of the lower legs. Visualize those muscles limp and loose. Continue in this manner until you reach your head. Then see all the muscles in your head relaxing. The muscles in the top of the head, your ears, eyelids, nose, jaws, tongue, etc.

As you practice the exercise you will find that it takes less and less time to develop a wonderful feeling of relaxation. Eventually, you will be able to relax instantly by just using the key words "RELAX NOW." It is important that you follow the instructions as given in the SEMANTIC-RELAXATION exercise. The words "RELAX NOW" will become a symbol that will trigger the response of total relaxation under any circumstances

If you learn nothing else than how to relax, your time will have been well spent. You will have learned how to do something you can use in any tense situation when relaxing will allow you to function with maximum effectiveness. However, there is much, much more you can achieve by learning how to write and give yourself auto-suggestion in this relaxed state. You will find all the information you need to make any changes in your life that you desire at this site. It is yours to use or not to use, as you choose. It will not cost you any money, but it is not totally free. Like anything worth learning, it does take time and commitment on your part.

HYPNOSIS AND CONDITIONING

This course in hypnosis is based on the Pavlovian science of reflex therapy. The scientific method is naturalistic. There are no supernatural phenomena presented here. It is our belief that all hypnotic phenomena are traceable to natural causes. Pavlov's fundamental experiments with dogs are well established. What is less well known is that the same principles of conditioning are equally applicable to human beings. It has been demonstrated that words can become the "bells" that trigger conditioned reflexes. Within the conditioned reflex is the essence of hypnosis. Pavlov suggested this when he wrote, "Speech, on account of the whole preceding life of the adult, is connected up with all the internal and external stimuli which can reach the cortex, signaling all of those reactions of the organism which are normally determined by the actual stimuli themselves. We can, therefore, regard 'suggestion' as the most simple form of a typical conditioned reflex in man."

There is never anything wrong with an individuals "should" department. Everyone knows what he should do. The problem is in the "able to" department. This is because we do not control ourselves. We are constantly controlled by our conditioned habit patterns. Our habits control our thoughts. Our emotional training determines our thinking. We only have the volition our habits allow us to have. If we have been conditioned to respond in a certain way, there is no free will. If an individual's learned reflexes are inadequate, he will bemoan his lack of "guts," and criticize himself, though he is not at all to blame. As intelligent as a human being may be, he can no more think his way out of an emotional problem than a jackass. He can only be trained out of it. We do not act because of intelligent reasons. Our reasons for acting are born in our emotional habits. It is important to realize that conditioning is not an intellectual process. Like it or not, the brain has been permeated by the viscera. The vast majority of what we do is done without thinking. This is also to our benefit, life would be impossible if we had to think to breathe, digest, feel, blink, maintain our balance, and keep our hearts beating.

Using self-hypnosis and auto-suggestion you can replace undesirable conditioned reflexes with desirable ones. Start by changing some minor problem that is not to difficult to change. Once you succeed, this will give you more confidence in yourself to try to replace a more difficult response with a desirable one.

WHAT IS HYPNOSIS?

There is really nothing strange or mysterious about the phenomenon of hypnosis. It is simply a particular state-of-mind that occurs quite naturally and spontaneously in each and every normal human being. In fact, you have experienced hypnosis to some degree every single day of your life. Each time that you have been totally absorbed in reading a favorite book, watching an interesting movie, daydreaming, or any number of similar situations, you have spontaneously entered into a hypnoidal state. During the time you remain in such a state, outside distractions no longer compete for your attention and you are better able to absorb those thoughts and ideas that you select as having special meaning for you.

Modern hypnotism is assumed to begin with the work of Franz Anton Mesmer, a Viennese physician. During the last half of the 18th century, Mesmer began developing a theory that he called "animal magnetism." Unfortunately, Mesmer's work took place during a time when fear and superstition hung over Europe like a dark cloud. Mesmerism, as it was called then, was looked upon as sorcery and witchcraft.

In the mid 1800's a Scottish physician by the name of James Braid scoffed at the idea of Mesmerism being sorcery or witchcraft. Braid believed that hypnosis was a special state of sleep that he referred to as "sleep of the nervous system." He coined the term "HYPNOSIS" after the Greek god of sleep, "Hypnos."

Today, we know that hypnosis is really not a sleep state. Through the use of sophisticated scientific instrumentation it has been shown that a hypnotized person is neither unconscious nor asleep. In fact, experiments using electroencephalographs to measure brain wave patterns have revealed that brain activity during hypnosis is often indistinguishable from that of persons engaged in normal mental activity.

Hypnotism gained real fame during World War II when many psychotherapists turned toward hypnotism in an attempt to find an effective method of dealing with "battle fatigue" and "war neuroses." Owing to its great success, hypnotism began to find wide acceptance by the medical profession. On April 23, 1955, hypnotism was officially recognized by the British Medical Association as a valid method of treatment. In September of 1958 the American Medical Association approved the use of hypnosis in medicine based on the favorable results of a long and intensive committee study of the subject.

The American Medical Association defines hypnosis as "a temporary condition of altered attention, within which a variety of phenomena may appear spontaneously or manifest themselves in response to verbal or other stimuli." To state it more simply, when a person is hypnotized, his ability to respond to suggestion is increased.

Hypnosis is generally associated with a state of complete relaxation. This special state of relaxation is one that you can, with practice, learn to create yourself. In this relaxed state, your mind is free to accept positive thoughts and ideas much more readily, enabling you to change fixed negative ideas into strong positive attitudes about yourself and your surroundings.

Hypnosis is a state that the individual actually creates within himself and each person experiences it in a unique way. Some experience the relaxation as a heavy sensation, others experience it as a light or tingling feeling and some experience no unusual sensation whatsoever and are only aware of its presence by the manner in which they are able to respond to suggestion. Some persons quite naturally respond with more intensity than do others. Many will enter the hypnotic state in a matter of seconds, while others may take considerably longer.

Highly resistant individuals may have any one of a number of reasons for not readily entering into the hypnotic state while following directions of the hypnotist. Fear is sometimes an obstacle -- fear based on false expectations. However, as the fearful individual gains more and more experience and awareness of the hypnotic state, his fears gradually disappear and he finds that each successive time he is able to enter into the state much more quickly, easily and deeply and with practice can achieve the same degree of success as the best hypnotic subject.

HYPNOSIS: FACTS AND FICTION

FICTION: A hypnotist is an unusual person gifted with some mysterious power of the mind.

FACT: The hypnotist does not possess any unusual or mysterious powers of the mind. He is a person very much like yourself, except that he understands certain aspects of the human mind that are not known to most people. He has also learned to master the art of suggestion which he uses to guide the individual toward developing greater awareness and control of the hypnotic state.

FICTION: Only gullible or weak-minded persons respond favorably to hypnosis.

FACT: Studies conducted at Stanford University have shown that intelligence is not an important factor in determining an individual's ability to respond favorably to hypnosis. Although, statistically, there is some evidence to indicate that persons with higher intelligence and greater creative abilities tend to be somewhat more responsive to suggestion.

FICTION: Hypnosis is dangerous.

FACT: In spite of scare articles in newspapers and magazines, there has not been one documented case of hypnosis doing harm to a person. There is no evidence that hypnosis will weaken the will, damage the nervous system, or in any other way adversely affect the physical and mental well-being of an individual. Research studies at Loyola University have shown that volunteer students hypnotized over 400 times experienced no adverse effects. On the contrary, there is some evidence to indicate that the hypnotic state is one in which the entire body tends to become self-regulating and functions with maximum efficiency. Some psychological disorders seem to correct themselves in hypnosis, even though no suggestions to that effect are given.

FICTION: To be hypnotized means being put to sleep and being completely unconscious of your surroundings.

FACT: Hypnosis is not sleep and there is definitely no loss of consciousness at any time. The hypnotized individual is always aware of what is occurring; in fact, his awareness actually increases.

FICTION: There have been cases where people have been unable to awaken from hypnosis.

FACT: A hypnotized person is not asleep; therefore, there should never be any concern about the person not awakening. Reports of persons remaining in the hypnotic state are exaggerated stories having no validity. The hypnotic state can always be terminated easily and quickly by the hypnotist or the individual.

FICTION: While in a deep hypnotic state, an individual may reveal intimate secrets or embarrassing details about himself.

FACT: During hypnosis the individual is always conscious (unlike with chemical anesthetics or truth serums) and aware of everything that is occurring. Therefore, in the same manner that he guards his secrets while awake, he also protects his secrets while hypnotized.

FICTION: In hypnosis you will blindly obey every command, good or bad.

FACT: In hypnosis the individual retains his ability to make judgments; therefore, he would never accept any command nor obey any order that he considers to be against his own best interests or contrary to his morals.

FICTION: A person must be placed in a very deep hypnotic state before hypnosis can be of any value to him.

FACT: Eighty-to-ninety percent of the work in hypnosis is accomplished in the light-to medium stages of hypnosis.

FICTION: Hypnosis always affects a change in just one or two sessions.

114

FACT: This has been true in many cases, but in general, a great number of sessions are usually required before complete results are obtained.

IS HYPNOSIS DANGEROUS?

Dr. Julius Grinker states, "The so-called dangers from hypnosis are imaginary. Although I have hypnotized many hundreds of patients, I have never seen any ill effects from its use."

Dr. David Cheek, M.D., who has vast experience in the field writes, "We can do more harm with ignorance of hypnotism than we can ever do by intelligently using hypnosis and suggestion constructively."

Psychologist Rafael Rhodes in his book "Therapy Through Hypnosis" writes "Hypnotism is absolutely safe. There is no known case on record of harmful results from its therapeutic use."

In his book, "Clinical and Experimental Hypnosis," Dr. William S. Kroger states, "Platonof, an associate of Pavlov, who used hypnosis over fifty years on over fifty-thousand cases, reports as follows: 'We have never observed any harmful influences on the patient which could be ascribed to the method of hypno-suggestion therapy, or any tendency toward the development of unstable personality, weakening of the will, or pathological urge for hypnosis. "

Dr. Louie P. Thorpe, Professor Emeritus, University of Southern California, in his book "The Psychology of Mental Health," writes, "Hypnotism is a natural phenomena, and there are no known deleterious effects from its use."

Leslie N. LeCron, psychologist and authority on hypnosis, states, "As to self-induction, many thousands have learned it; and I have yet to hear a report of any bad results of its use."

Andre M. Weitzenhoffer, Ph.D., a highly respected authority in the field of hypnotism writes, "As far as it is known today, hypnosis per se is no more dangerous than natural sleep. There is no evidence that hypnosis in itself weakens the will, damages the nervous system, or in any way adversely affects the mental and physical well-being of individuals."

IDEOMOTOR ACTION

Human thought manifests itself in two forms. We can think using visual images or by using words (language). Language consists of sound symbols used as a means of communication between two individuals. Objects in the exterior world are designated by sound symbols that permits them to be envisioned even in their absents. However, words become detached from the objects they symbolize and take on an independent life. They no longer are only a means of communication, but become an instrument of thought. Words become an internal language, which is no longer speech, since it is not expressed in sound, but a method of thinking.

115

No matter which method we use for thinking, the end result is a change in the musculature of our body. If you think of performing some act, the muscles of your body responsible for carrying out that act are enervated whether you actually carry out the act or not. If you think about buttoning your shirt, or describe how to button a shirt to someone else, the muscles of your body that would be used to perform the action are energized and in an aborted way carry out the act. This is why the Semantic-Relaxation Exercise works. If you suggest to yourself or imagine that a muscle or groups of muscles are relaxing, they actually respond to some small degree. Through repetition the response becomes greater and more generalize. I don't expect you to believe this. I intend to let you perform a little experiment and prove it to yourself. For the experiment you will need a piece of string or thread and a small weight of some kind (i.e., heavy button, bead about 3/4" in diameter, etc.).

Attach your weight (button etc.) to the string as illustrated above. What we are creating is just a pendulum, a small bob hanging to a thread or string. Almost any small object will do. The dimensions given are not critical. If you use a button it should be about 3/8 to ½ inch in diameter. The color is unimportant. What you will have created, if you decide to make the object above, is called Chevreul's pendulum.

This experiment can be performed while you are in any comfortable position. Just hold the end of the string so that the weighted end can swing freely. One way to do it is to sit at a table. Rest your left forearm in your lap or along the edge of the table. Rest your right elbow with your right arm lifted almost vertically, a little forward of your left arm. Hold the end of the string between your finger and thumb. Position yourself so that you are comfortable. If you are sitting as described, the pendulum should hang in front of the center of your body (median plane). The bob should be about ½ " from the top of the table. Actually none of these instructions are crucial, if you approximate them the experiment is virtually certain to succeed.

After you have assumed your position, the bob will probably be swinging freely in some direction. With your left hand bring it to a stand still (if you are left handed, reverse hands). Put your hand back into position. If the pendulum is not perfectly still don't worry about it, its not that important. Now fix your gaze on the bob and imagine that it is the pendulum on a grandfather's clock. Imagine that it is swinging from side-to-side just like a pendulum on a clock. The more you can see the pendulum swinging from side to side in your imagination, the greater the response will be. Follow with your eyes an imaginary pendulum on a clock moving from side to side. Try not to think about anything else and do not try to analyze what is happening. If you followed the above instructions, the pendulum will do exactly what you imagine.

Once you have the pendulum swinging from side to side, without stopping it, imagine that the bob is sitting on the edge of a phonograph record and the record is going around and around. As you imagine the bob going around on the outer edge of the disk, you will find that the side to side motion changes into a rotary motion. Once the bob starts going in circles, imagine that the record is spinning faster and faster. The bob will begin to make a larger circle and pick up speed.

Some individuals when first trying this experiment tend to tense their muscles. This should not be done and will only serve to lessen the response. Try to be relaxed when you try this experiment. The only people that this experiment will not work for are those individuals that "know" before they start, it will not work. However, if they are thinking, "this will not work, the bob will not move." The experiment is working for them, they are getting exactly what they are thinking. "the bob will not move" and it will not.

The Chevreul pendulum experiment is a demonstration of the phenomenon of ideomotor action. That is, the tendency of thoughts or ideas to be automatically translated, reflex like, into specific patterns of muscular activity. Probably many hypnotic suggestions act purely through ideomotor action. As stimuli they trigger corresponding thoughts and images that act as cue-producing responses, evoking actual motor responses. The repeated elicitation of an ideomotor response increases the intensity of the response.

Ideomotor actions tend to be weak responses, particularly in their initial phrase. If there is present another strong muscular action or tension involving the same muscles it will tend to mask or block the weak pattern induced by thoughts. The probabilities are that you will succeed with this experiment as very few people fail to get a response. If you do not get any results, do not give up. Try again on several consecutive days or try using a lighter or heaver bob. You might try a different length of string. In general, a longer string will give a greater response.

If you have performed the experiment as outlined above, you should begin to understand why the Semantic-Relaxation Exercise works. Instead of imagining that a pendulum is swinging, we imagine that all the muscles in our body are relaxing. This is exactly what happens. At first the response to our suggestions of relaxation are weak, but with repetition they become more and more effective. The relaxation becomes greater and occurs more quickly. As a result of the "voluntary" muscles relaxing, the viscera, including the heart, blood vessels and other internal organs relax. It has been clinically demonstrated that if you relax your skeletal muscles, the internal muscles tend to relax also.

INSTRUCTIONS FOR THE SEMANTIC-IMAGERY RELAXATION EXERCISE

(A slow but sure way to enter the hypnotic state)

To Induce A State Of Self-Relaxation, Follow These Instructions Carefully:

Select a comfortable location where you can be sure that you will not be distracted by the telephone or other unnecessary noises or interruptions.

Subdued lighting and a quiet atmosphere are helpful but not essential. The area should be free from drafts and unpleasant odors.

Clothing should be loose (tie, belt, shoes, etc.).

You may do this exercise sitting up or lying down, whichever is more convenient.

If you are seated, make sure that your back is supported against the back of the chair. Feet should be flat on the floor, or use a footrest. Knees and ankles should not be crossed. Hands should rest on the arms of the chair or on your thighs or loosely on your lap. The head should be in a comfortable forward position.

If you are lying down, your arms should be alongside your body and your head should be slightly elevated. Feet should be separated with toes turned outward.

Set a time limit for your practice session. Initially, you may want to use a timer to signal you when the time is up. With practice you will learn to respond accurately to your own internal clock.

STEP 1: Locate an imaginary spot on the ceiling or the wall. Focus your attention on the imaginary spot and remain perfectly still.

STEP 2: Vividly imagine that you feel calm, relaxed and sleepy. Your body responds to your imagination and the more you pretend, the more your body will respond.

STEP 3: As you begin to feel your eyelids becoming heavy, take three deep breaths.

After the first deep breath, slowly exhale and say or think..."I am relaxing."

After the second deep breath, slowly exhale and say or think..."My body is relaxing."

On the third deep breath, hold it and count..."Three...two...one." Then as you exhale, say or think the words, "RELAX NOW" and let your eyelids close.

STEP 4: Direct your attention to each group of muscles in your body and tell them to relax. In your imagination, see them relaxing. Start at the tips of your toes and continue to the top of your head.

Do this exercise slowly and without concern. Allow 10 to 15 minutes for the body to relax. DO NOT test the relaxation by moving.

STEP 5: At the end of each practice session think to yourself..."Each time I practice this exercise I relax more quickly, more easily and more deeply than any time before. Each time I am more receptive and responsive to suggestions I give to myself. I look forward to practicing daily because I enjoy it."

STEP 6: Slowly count from 1 to 5 to arouse yourself. Before counting, give yourself a suggestion that on the count of five you will be fully alert, feeling perfect in every way.

If you should have any concerns about arousing yourself at any time during your relaxation exercise, you will be reassured to know that you will always be aware of anything of significance that may be occurring at the time; and therefore, will always be in control of any unexpected situations that may arise.

If you are interrupted during a practice session, if possible, always take a moment to count from 1 to 5 before arousing.

Rules For Structuring Auto-Suggestions

1. REPETITION: This is the most important rule in making successful suggestions. A suggestion cannot be repeated too often. All advertising is based on suggestion, and advertisers know the value of repetition. Commercials of TV are repeated again and again, as you have undoubtedly noted with some annoyance.

A suggestion has the power to suppress or inhibit its reverse concept in the mind. Once a suggestion is conditioned in our nervous system, there is an impulse to carry it out immediately. That action temporarily bars any impulse to carry out the opposite impulse not to act, and vise versa.

2. BE POSITIVE: A suggestion is more likely to be accepted if it is characterized by a firm belief in the idea presented. Doubt seems to block results and negate the suggestion. You should think positively about it and feel sure the desired results will come. If you say, "I'll try," you are implying doubt. You really expect to fail and probably will. Your attitude should be that you are going to do it and not try. When you say, "I can't" you probably mean "I don't want to."

119

Eliminate every possible negative word. DO NOT mention what you are trying to move away from. Create a word picture of what you wish to move toward. If you suggest, "I am not self-conscious" you trigger the feeling of self-consciousness, and the memory of past experiences when you have felt self-conscious. Instead suggest, "I like people. I enjoy the company of people. When I am with people, I am calm, poised and relaxed.

RIGHT: "I sleep deeply, soundly, all night long."

WRONG: "I do not toss and turn for hours before going to sleep."

3. BE LOGICAL: A suggestion should be accurate and a sound reason given for its acceptance. For example, it is futile to eliminate a headache by suggesting: "Your headache is gone," for the subject feels the discomfort of the headache and knows it is there. Even in hypnosis, his first thought would be, "It is not gone, I still feel it." Most subjects would then reject the suggestion and the headache would continue. However, if we suggest, "Your headache will gradually lessen and in a few moments will be gone," it allows time for the suggestion to take place. If a logical reason is given why the headache will go away, the suggestion is almost certain to be accepted. For example, it can be suggested that his body is relaxed, he is resting and there is no longer a reason for the headache to remain.

If your desired result is one that can be measured, such as weight or a bowling score, suggest the exact improvement you desire. Some people seem to believe, if their ideal weight is 125 pounds, they can suggest they will lose weight until they reach 115 pounds. The idea being, if they are only partially successful they will still reach their goal. You cannot fool yourself. Suggest exactly what you want.

There are circumstances where it's wrong to suggest perfection. "I always organizes my time perfectly" is an impossibility for a mother of three children. "I am always enthusiastic" is a poor suggestion. Do you want to be enthusiastic at a funeral?

4. USE VISUAL IMAGES: A verbal suggestion will be more forceful if a visual image can be formed and added to it. Visual images will always aid the processes of conditioning. For example, if you are tired and wish to overcome this feeling by suggestion, visualize yourself doing something where you are active and full of energy. In your imagination see yourself playing golf or tennis. Carry this thought out for three or four minutes and the results can be quite surprising. Your visual images should always represent the desired end result.

5. USE EXCITING AND EMOTIONAL WORDS: It is well known that conditioning takes place very rapidly when we are experiencing some strong emotion. If a suggestion can be woven into some emotion, it is very beneficial. This may be by means of words or a visual image or both. Desire for

success can be such an emotion. Use such words as: vibrant, sparkling, thrilling, wonderful, powerful, radiant, loving, generous, exciting, delightful and beautiful.

6. BE SIMPLE: Be sure your wording says what you mean and is not ambiguous. Use simple language. Avoid long technical terms and psychological or metaphysical phrases. This is not a thesis you are writing for a professor to score. Simple words have the greatest force. Ernest Hemingway became famous for the simplicity of his writing, yet it had a tremendous impact.

7. USE PRESENT TENSE: Always, when ever possible, phrase your suggestions as though they were already an accomplished fact. Even suggestions for future behavior should be given in the present tense. For example, "Next Thursday when I stand to speak at the company dinner, I am calm, poised and relaxed." Suggestions phrased in the future become another "New Years resolution" easy to forget and not taken seriously.

Never refer to past conditions in your suggestions. This brings a dual image into your mind, the image of how you have been and how you wish to be. Naturally the image of how you have been is the stronger of the two. An exception to this rule is when you are dealing with a physical condition, such as a broken leg. The progressive form of the present tense is used to bypass the critical factor of your logical mind. "Each day my leg grows stronger and healthier." If you were to say, "My leg is strong and healthy" your logical mind would reject the suggestion.

RIGHT: I am...It is...I feel...

WRONG: I will...It will...I am going to...

8. BE SPECIFIC: Choose one specific area for self-improvement and confine your efforts to that area. Do not give yourself suggestions for two or three problems all at the same time. You can work on more than one problem by alternating your suggestions. Work with repetition on one suggestion for two or three sessions then change to another. Do not suggest that you are filled with confidence, sleep perfectly every night, wear a size twelve dress, express love to your children and have given up cigarettes. Work on one goal until you feel some change, then move on to another. You may get results with your first suggestion, many people do, but be prepared to use the same suggestion once a day for two weeks before moving on to your next goal.

9. BE DETAILED: Analyze your goal and structure your suggestion to cover every detail of your desired change of behavior.

RIGHT: "I like people. I enjoy being with people. People are aware that I like them and they return the feeling. I especially enjoy talking to people when I stand before an audience; I want to do things for them. I feel a wave of friendship and understanding flowing from every member of the audience to me. As I begin speaking my lips are flexible, my mouth is moist, I breathe deeply from the diaphragm. My legs are strong beneath me. My hands are poised and calm. The gestures flow spontaneously and freely. I have the undivided attention of the audience and it makes me feel secure and confident. There is a smile in my heart, which comes to my lips at the proper times. I speak easily, freely and confidently. I speak with a full release of my knowledge, skill and ability. When my talk is concluded, I am gratified by the applause."

WRONG: I will be an excellent public speaker.

10. PERSONALIZE: Structure your suggestions to change yourself, your attitudes, your actions. Don't suggestion a change in others. As you change those associated with you change. Try to describe your actions rather than your abilities.

RIGHT: "My family and my friends co-operate with me because I am interested in their welfare."

WRONG: "My children always respect and obey me."

RIGHT: "I take a sincere and enthusiastic interest in my children, their friends and I understand their point of view. I express love and approval of my children. It is easy for me to express my love for them."

One thing to keep in mind is that suggestions can and do work both ways. Negative suggestions can also be effective. We are constantly bombarded with suggestions. An unpleasant trick can be played on an individual in an office by using negative suggestions. When he arrives in the morning a fellow worker greets him with the remark, "Good heavens, Tom, you must have had a bad night. You really look terrible this morning." Tom has been feeling quite well and is surprised at this statement. A few minutes later someone remarks casually, "Got a hangover this morning, Tom? You sure look bad." Another inquires sympathetically if he has a fever. By this time Tom is feeling poorly and any further repetition is likely to send him home actually ill.

One important part of self-therapy is to locate and dehypnotize yourself of negative and detrimental suggestions that may be affecting you. We all carry these suggestions with us and are generally unaware of them.

Rules for Applying Auto-Suggestions

1. WRITE out your suggestion following the rules you have been given (see Rules For Structuring Auto-Suggestions). Writing forces us to crystallize our ideas. It makes us analyze the problem that we are facing, and is an aid to clear thinking.

2. SYMBOLIZE your suggestion. Find a key or code word that symbolizes the feeling and content of your suggestion. Select a simple word, if possible that means to you the entire suggestion. For example, a suggestion designed to help a person to overcome feelings of inferiority could be symbolized by the word "Confidence." Finding the correct symbol is extremely important. The symbol doesn't have to mean a thing to anyone else; it is for you and should cause a strong surge of feeling or create a picture for you.

3. EDIT your suggestion. Read the written suggestion to make sure it complies with the rules. Revise it. Reconstruct it. Expand it. Condense it. Recopy the revised version and destroy the first copy.

4. READ your suggestion aloud before hypnotizing yourself. When in the presents of others where reading might be embarrassing or impossible, the suggestion can be read silently but very carefully. Reading aloud is much preferable because it forces us to verbalize every word. When reading silently we have a tendency to skip and scan. In a properly edited suggestion, every word is important.

5. HYPNOTIZE yourself. Use the master key method; "RELAX NOW," etc.

6. THINK the symbol. As soon as you feel the onset of deep relaxation, whisper or think the symbol to yourself. Make no effort to remember the wording of your suggestion. By reading your suggestion before hypnotizing yourself you have given yourself a pre- hypnotic suggestion. You have so to speak, loaded the gun. When you think the symbol, you are pulling the trigger on a loaded gun. Certain phrases from your suggestion will drift into your mind, as they do, create a feeling response to the words. Visualize yourself acting in the way you wish to act, feeling the way you wish to feel and successfully doing the things you want to do.

To make a dramatic change in your life or to overcome deep-seated un-adaptive habits, it is necessary to structure a detailed suggestion, symbolize it and use the above technique to make it work.

The reason for the pre-suggestion, symbolization and trigger release, is that as you go into the hypnotic state your conscious, analytical mind slows down. If you try to remember long suggestions or form new detailed suggestions, you tend to lighten the hypnotic state. By just using the symbol, you release the entire concept with a minimum of conscious activity.

PROCEDURES FOR DEEPENING THE HYPNOTIC TRANCE

If you have been practicing the techniques and procedures for inducting the hypnotic state, you should at this point be able to achieve complete physical relaxation in about fifteen minutes or less. Now you should begin to practice attaining this relaxation without mentally going over your whole body area by area. After you have taken the three breaths and said mentally, "Relax now," give yourself this suggestion: "My entire body is loose, limp and relaxed." Now visualize or imagine any picture that means to you complete physical relaxation (a rag doll or a hand full of loose rubber bands, etc.). Some people get perfect results by remembering the sensation they have while practicing semantic relaxation. It is important to learn to produce this state of relaxation quickly so that you can move to the techniques for deepening your state of hypnosis, testing for depth, and programming new mental responses.

DEEPENING TECHNIQUES

One of the most elementary yet effective methods of increasing trance depth is simply to suggest, each time you practice, that you will go deeper the next time. This usually has an additive effect, and if you get into the habit of including this thought along with any other suggestion concept, you may be surprised to find, when you get to the point of testing, that you are going deeper than you had realized.

Another technique is to use one of the counting methods. As soon as you feel your body begin to relax, start counting backward from one hundred in this manner: "One hundred, deeper asleep, ninety-nine, deeper asleep," and so on. The moment that you are not sure what number you thought last, "was it eighty three or eighty two," stop counting, you are now in deep hypnosis. At this point your mind has slowed down, but still able to function with little effort. This is the depth of hypnosis where you can feel an emotional response to your positive suggestions and mental pictures.

Try not to analyze or evaluate your depth of hypnosis at this point. Use any conscious energy you have at the time to think of positive concepts you wish to achieve. Remember, as you go deeper your ability to evaluate is diminished. In a way you become less "aware," even of your decreased "awareness."

Another variation of the counting method is to picture yourself writing 100 on a blackboard. Then mentally erase the 100 and write "deeper asleep" off to one side; then write 99 and so on until you are not sure what number is next.

Another good technique is to picture in your imagination that you are riding backward down an escalator. As you are slowly drifting down, picture a red neon sign at the top of the staircase. The sign is flashing, "deeper asleep"... "deeper asleep." As you go farther and farther down, the sign becomes smaller and more indistinct.

Remember, the goal that you are working toward is NOT sleep. You are learning to achieve a state of self-hypnosis in which you are physically, and mentally relaxed to a day-dreamy like state. Your conscious mind is still functioning, but not in a rapid, alert and analytical way it functions when you are awake. This mental state is one in which your powers of visualization are increased, your feeling response is greater, and your critical powers are diminished, but not totally absent.

Note: Whenever you use imagery, try to think or imagine, SUBJECTIVELY rather than objectively. See the things and scenes themselves, rather than seeing yourself seeing them.

TESTING THE HYPNOTIC TRANCE

The only purpose of testing is to satisfy yourself as to the depth of self-hypnosis that you have reached. Some people never use tests because they easily learn to recognize the "feeling" of hypnosis and do not question or worry about depth. If you are one of those fortunate people and already realize that you have achieved self-hypnosis, do not waste time on tests. Use this time to program your nervous system with positive ideas and mental pictures. If you are still having trouble recognizing the "feeling" of hypnosis, the tests will prove to you that you are hypnotizing yourself.

There are several tests that we have used in our classes that you can give yourself. They are the handclasp, arm-rigidity, arm levitation and eye catalepsy tests. You can easily re-create these at home.

The eye catalepsy test is done as follows: After hypnotizing yourself, picture two windows with the shades drawn. Then visualize that the springs in the rollers have lost their tension and therefore it is impossible to raise the shades. When you have a good picture of this, imagine that your eyes are the windows, and your eyelids are the window shades, then relax the muscles in the eyelids so much that they would not work if you wanted them to. When you KNOW that you have relaxed them that much, roll your eyeballs up in your head as if you were going to look out a hole in your forehead, now say, "My eyelids are so relaxed they just won't work," then try to open your eyes. Now, when we say try to open your eyes, we do NOT mean that you should try and keep on trying, because if you struggle long enough you lighten your state of hypnosis. Just give a brief try and when the thought comes, "good heavens they're really stuck," RELAX, stop trying.

The handclasp test is given in this manner: Clasp your hands together tightly and extend your arms out in front of yourself with your elbows straight. Now imagine a strong rope being looped around your arms at the elbows in such a manner that it draws the elbows toward each other. Now imagine that there is a strong liquid glue being poured over your hands and that it is drying hard and sticking your hands together into one solid mass. Think about the rope around your arms being drawn even tighter. Develop this to the point where your arms are strained and stiff. Think again of the glue as now being hard and solid around your hands. Keep this in mind as you go back once more to the rope. When you are imagining the rope vividly as getting tighter, you can try hard to take your hands apart, but you will be unable to do so. Let the thought go through your mind that the harder you try, the more firmly your hands are stuck together. You will find this is so!

Arm-rigidity test: After hypnotizing yourself, extend your arm straight out in front of you. Curl the fingers of that hand into a tight fist. Now imagine your arm as if it were carved out of wood and sticking straight out in front of you stiff and rigid! Keep thinking of your arm this way -- stiff and rigid. Now, imagine that you are writing the word "rigid" on the blackboard and that each time you write the word "rigid" your arm gets stiffer. See your arm so stiff and rigid that you cannot bend it. See yourself trying to bend your arm but the more you try the stiffer it becomes. After a few seconds tell yourself to relax and let your arm drop to your side.

This is the way you give yourself the arm levitation test at home: Hypnotize yourself and give yourself this suggestion; "I am going to count to ten, as I do a pleasant feeling of lightness moves into my hand and arm, as I continue counting my fingers begin to lift and move, then my hand begins to lift and finally my arm begins to lift and continues rising until it is touching my face. Imagine as clearly as you can a balloon tied to your wrist with a piece of strong string. Imagine that this is a big balloon filled with gas and it is so light it is pulling your arm up. Now begin counting to ten. With each count imagine another balloon is being tied to your arm. Develop this image clearly. Think about the color of the balloons being tied to your arm, think about their size and shape. As each balloon is tied to your wrist feel the pull of the balloons increasing. At the count of ten as the last balloon is tied to your arm, think of your arm floating up, higher and higher. Do NOT try to resist. This is not a contest, you could resist if you chose to, but that is not the purpose of the test.

ADDITIONAL INSTRUCTIONS

Once you have started to give yourself a test, avoid analyzing or thinking of anything else. Practice the tests with the attitude, ambiguous, as it may seem, of not caring whether or not you get results. This is far more effective than an intensive effort to succeed. Over anxiety in any form is apt to be inhibitive. In the beginning, do not keep trying to open your eyes or separating your hands for more than a few seconds. Although it is important for you to experience this difficulty, remember it is not caused by some external force but by responses developed by your own mental processes. This is what you want to happen as a step to more important accomplishments. Except the response of your hands feeling stuck together or your eyelids stuck together for a few seconds as evidence of your effective use of suggestion and imagery in bringing about a physiological reaction.

You are learning that you must separate the conditioning of a response from the testing of the response. If during the conditioning or suggesting procedure you are thinking about whether or not it is going to work, this will lessen the effectiveness of the conditioning. If on the other hand, you "know" it is going to be successful, this will help to make it so. The systematic compounding of one belief, held even temporarily, upon another leads to conviction. It is conviction that we are seeking here.

Your attitude is a major factor in achieving good results. Each time something happens in a satisfactory way, you should let the success build confidence and belief in your ability and in the technique you are using. Magnify this in your mind as much as you can. Try to minimize any lack of response and simply think, "It will happen soon and will then be a better response than if it had happened too quickly."

The proper degree of cooperation is important. This does NOT mean that you should just go ahead and perform the response consciously. It means that you should act "as if" the imagined situation were actually in existence and as if the response were actually occurring because of existing circumstances.

Mentally prepare yourself for self hypnosis -- think; "Now I am going to hypnotize myself." NOT "Well I suppose I better try to hypnotize myself, it probably won't work, I'm not one of the lucky ones." This is a NEGATIVE autosuggestion! A reluctance to practice or a negative attitude about your ability to hypnotize yourself may indicate a reluctance to assume responsibility for your own life.

If you find that you fall asleep when you practice self-hypnosis do NOT practice after you are in bed for the night. Practice during the day or early evening and use the floor, an easy chair or couch. Do NOT practice self-hypnosis behind the wheel of your car; instead get in the back seat or move over to the passenger's side.

Don't panic if you are not getting results as fast as some. Take it easy, do not pressure yourself; let your fears fade away at the speed to which you can adjust. "Slow" students invariably find once they have stopped trying so hard they suddenly have progressed to a more advanced stage without realizing it. Remember, EVERYONE IS HYPNOTIZABLE.

EMOTIONAL BEHAVIOR

EMOTION IS A PECULIAR WORD. Almost everyone uses it and thinks he knows what it means until he attempts to define it. Emotion is many things for many people. For some it is a mental experience; for others it is a way of acting; for many it is a series of events occurring within their bodies. Some regard most emotion as "bad," while others regard much emotion as "good."

Those who consider most emotion as bad would probably say we should understand and study it in order to minimize the disruptive influence it has on our lives. They might point out that during such emotions as rage or fear we act irrational and our judgment becomes impaired. This is true, we would have to agree with them, sometimes emotion may do us harm and we therefore should attempt to control it.

Those that consider most emotion as good would probably point out that unemotional people are either dull or "cold-blooded" and calculating. They would claim it enriches our lives by removing apathy and motivates us to learn and plan our lives. We would have to agree with them, as we know that anxieties for the future cause us to plan our lives. We also know, excitement, fear or rage gives us strength for acts that we ordinarily could not accomplish.

Regardless of how we think of emotion or what we think it is almost everyone considers it important to life. Recently there has been another reason for impressing the importance of emotion on us. It is the growing realization by modern medicine that many of our diseases -- whether called "mental" or physical -- are intimately related to emotion. It is now well known that any strong emotion results in a vast complex of internal changes that involve muscular, chemical, glandular and neural activity throughout the entire body. In fact it is the physiological aspects of emotion that distinguish it most clearly from other psychological processes.

It has been long common to regard the neuroses and the psychoses as associated with preceding extreme emotion. More recently science has discovered that a host of ailments termed PSYCHOSOMATIC DISORDERS (i.e., asthma, high blood pressure, and many skin ailments) are associated with emotion. Regardless of whether we consider emotion as good or bad, we cannot escape the conclusion that emotional behavior is important in everyday life.

During the eighteen hundreds man began to become aware of the importance of the brain. It was generally believed that the brain was the "seat" of the emotions. Today science has shown that emotion is more physical than mental. Emotion is considered a psycho-physiological response. In other words, what we are conscious of, as emotion is the sensation caused by a response pattern occurring in our viscera, glands and skeletal muscles.

Take the emotion fear for example. Fear presents many physiological symptoms as it varies from "apprehension" to "terror." Many of the physiological patterns of fear are well known. How often have you heard the term "cold feet," used to describe cowardice? Cold hands and paleness are also well known symptoms of fear. Slightly less obvious and less well recognized physiological characteristics of fear are dry mouth and wide eyes. That "lump-in-the-stomach" reaction to fear is an inhibition of peristalsis (muscular action of the intestines). One other well-known reaction is tenseness of the skeletal muscles.

Anger causes other physiological symptoms. There is an increase in the amount of adrenaline and sugar in the blood. Sweat breaks out all over the body. The temperature of the skin may rise or fall several degrees. Again the skeletal muscles become very tense.

The emotion embarrassment involves still other physical reactions. One of the characteristic signs of embarrassment is blushing, or vasodilatation, in the head and neck regions. We might point out the fact that you use this response as your real criterion for judging the presence or absence of embarrassment.

One last example is disgust or revulsion. If this emotion is strong enough it can cause reverse peristalsis in the gastro-intestinal tract (vomiting). You have probably heard the expression, "It was so disgusting I wanted to vomit."

During and following almost any kind of increased emotional activity the tone of the skeletal muscles increase. What we call "emotional tension" is really our awareness of muscle tension. The more tense our skeletal muscles become, the more emotional we become. On the other hand, as we "discharge" or reduce our muscular tension we reduce emotion. This fact gives us a key to reducing or eliminating emotional behavior we do not want.

There are probably some of you that feel "emotion" is mental rather than a physical response. We wish to emphasize that we have no desire to minimize its importance in emotional behavior. We only wish to get emotion per se "out of the mind." That we all are aware of and experience emotion is unquestionable. That we become aware of external stimuli that trigger feeling of satisfaction or annoyance is obvious. That we perceive certain visceral events (i.e., stomach cramp or fast heart beat) and report them as "feelings" is also clear. What we want to emphasize is that we vaguely perceive certain other visceral, glandular and muscular changes and report them as feelings of anger, affection, annoyance, delight, dejection, depression, disgust, elation, embarrassment, fear, happiness, jealousy, shame, worry, and so on. We also wish to point out that when one uses such words to describe a change in "feeling" when there are no muscular and visceral changes present, then there is not a change in emotion. Such reactions are ideational in nature and lack a perception or feeling of change. Many of our so-called "pleasures" or "displeasures" are solely mental reactions. For example, we say we are "happy" about something, or displeased" at something else. We say we "hate" to lose a bet, or that we love our country or dog. Most such verbal reports are expressions of attitudes or ideas. With out muscular, visceral and glandular changes they are not reflections of emotion. Accompanied with muscular, visceral and glandular changes, they represent a mental concurrent quality of emotion.

It is universally recognized that muscle tension is the most common symptom of most emotional states. These muscular tensions tend to become habitual and often persist even after there is no outward evidence of emotional behavior or feeling. Embarrassments long forgotten, childhood failures and ancient disappointments, frustrations and fears that lie buried beneath the level of consciousness, persist and continue to torture us. They persist mainly in our habits of muscular tensions. Many people become accustomed to these chronic tensions and consider them normal. That many of us suffer from chronic tension is shown by the tens of millions of tranquilizers that are sold in this country every year.

The signs of chronic tension are varied. Some individuals may merely show indications of fatigue and added irritability. Some may appear to grow old, acquiring gray hair and added lines and folds in their face. Some become unable to fall asleep or else sleep through the night (there are also millions of sleeping pills sold in this country every year). The most common signs of emotional muscular tension are upsets in digestion. If accompanied by fever, diarrhea or vomiting, as often occurs, these upsets are likely to be attributed to something that was eaten. An over tense (spastic) digestive tract cannot properly digest food.

The question that interests us the most is, what do we do to alleviate these conditions? We have to start someplace. We must begin by learning how to relax and develop habit patterns of muscular relaxation. This is always the first step to health. Its importance cannot be over emphasized. Once you have learned to relax your voluntary muscles, a tremendous percentage of your emotional disturbances will disappear. You will automatically attain a large degree of tranquility and peace of mind. Many of your superficial neuroses and their associated physical symptoms will vanish.

The reason for this is simple. Emotional disturbances cause muscular tension, this in turn increases the emotional disturbance -- and around and around we go, winding up in the vortex of a deep depression. Once you learn to relax completely, there will be no anxiety impulses coming from any of your muscles to your brain. As a consequences, your brain and nervous system will also be relaxed and at ease. You will find yourself fully relaxed physically and mentally, at peace with the world and yourself.

Practicing the method of semantic relaxation, that we have given you, you will soon find that the depth of relaxation is so deep that ten to fifteen minutes will be equivalent to hours of ordinary sleep.

There is no doubt in my mind, if you learn nothing other than the technique of semantic relaxation in this course, you will have gained invaluable benefits. I do not ask you to believe a word of this, all I ask is that you give the idea a chance by practicing the technique, and see for yourself. Since physiological relaxation cannot be harmful and actually is as beneficial as any other hygienic practice, you have nothing to lose and everything to gain.

130

The method is called semantic relaxation because instead of trying to relax (trying is the opposite of relaxation) you will only verbally ask your muscles to relax and let nature take its course. After several weeks of practice, you will find by using the key symbol technique (relax now) you will be able to relax instantly and completely.

Each time you use this technique, you will find that your state of relaxation becomes deeper. You will find it a wonderful feeling. It is as though you were floating on a cloud, light as a feather, drifting effortlessly into a deeper and deeper state of relaxation. As your muscles relax, all tension and anxiety drop away. All worries disappear. You obtain relaxation of the mind and body to a degree that you never before dreamed possible.

Remember, as in most things, practice makes perfect. Repeat the exercises until you have mastered semantic relaxation completely. Then you will have taken a giant step toward freeing yourself from tension, toward a happier, healthier, and better life.

NEURO-DYNAMICS

As a submarine glides beneath the surface of the ocean, the only contact the crew has with the outside world is by way of instruments within the ship. The radar screen, sonic depth finder, radio receiver and other equipment tell the crew what is going on outside. This information is picked up by receptors, such as the radar and radio antennas located on the outer surface of the submarine.

As we move about in our environments, we function much as the submarine. This may seem wrong to you. For example, you may look across the way and see a red automobile. Actually this is not true. The automobile is not "red" and you do not "see" it. What takes place is this: All the light "falling" on the automobile is absorbed by the surface of the automobile, except the light we call red. The red light is reflected by the car. This reflected red light strikes your eye, resulting in an electro-chemical reaction in that sense organ. Neurons are excited which transmit electro-chemical messages to the visual centers of your brain. A neural pattern is set up that represents "red car."

In a similar way, you react to changes in your other sense organs and not to external objects. This may sound like "splitting hairs" to you, or you may feel its true, but so what. As we continue, you will see how important it is.

Sense organs, such as your eyes, ears, skin, etcetera that are found on the surface of your body are known a "receptors." They are "receivers" of information from the outside world. Each receptor is connected by a nerve to your high nervous system, the spinal cord and brain.

131

All around you is your environment; it is full of objects and people. They all affect you in some way. The person next to you may spill something on you, or she may give you a pleasant smile. These things that affect you are called "signals." The liquid spilled on you, is a signal. The pleasant smile is a signal.

A signal brings about a change in one or more of your receptors. The change in your receptors is called a "stimulus." This term is easy to remember because the change in your receptor "stimulates," or starts, a nerve impulse on its way to your brain.

As we encounter all kinds of stimulus situations, messages (nerve impulses) are received, evaluated, integrated and stored by our higher nervous system. Other messages in turn are sent out to various muscles and glands of your body. These muscles and glands are called "effectors." The change brought about in your effectors is called the "response."

All observable mental responses, without exception, can be reduced to a single phenomenon -- muscular movement. Whether its a child smiling at its mother, a young lady trembling at the first thought of love, or Isaac Newton discovering universal laws and writing them down on paper -- the ultimate reaction in all cases is muscular movement. But, you may say, most cerebral activity is expressed in words. But words are only combinations of sounds produced by muscular movements of the larynx and mouth cavity. Thus, all external manifestations of mental activity can be reduced to muscular movement.

This stimulus-response (S-R) action is the foundation of all your behavior. Everything you do is a matter of stimulus and response. Suppose you hear your name. The sound of your name (the signal) brings about a change (the stimulus) which sends a nerve impulse to your brain and on through your brain to your muscles. Your muscles (the effectors) then turn you toward the sound. This turning is the response.

If you bite into something good and ask for more, this is what takes place: The food (the signal) causes a change (the stimulus) in your tongue. The change (the stimulus) sends nerve impulses to and through your brain and out to your jaw, lips, lungs, and vocal muscles. These function to say the words, "Please give me some more." This is the response.

The action from stimulus to response is automatic. Most of what we do is done for us automatically. The majority of the business of living has little to do with what we call "thinking." In deciding to lift a cup of coffee, this is all we do consciously. The rest is done for us automatically by reflex action. We do not decide what muscles we need to use to lift the cup of coffee. We do not consciously regulate the exact degree of tension need by the muscles involved. All this is done for us at an unconscious level.

132

Your stimulus-response arcs account for all of your behavior. In order to form new responses or alter old ones, we must change our stimulus-response arcs. Ivan Pavlov was the first to make a scientific study of our stimulus-response arcs. In his original experiment it was found that a dog salivated as he ate meat, but did not salivate when a bell was rung. However, when the bell was rung just before the dog was fed, and this procedure was repeated a few times, an unexpected thing took place. The ringing of the bell alone could cause the dog to salivate. The sound of the bell had become the signal for food. In other experiments a square figure became the signal for a fear response or the flashing of a light became the signal for food.

It was also discovered that these signals tend to generalize. For example, if a square paired with a shock produced a fear response, a rectangle would also produce the same response.

From a physiological point of view what was happening is this: If some signal -- food or a chemical -- is brought into contact with the mouth a nerve impulse is transmitted by afferent nerves to a receiving center in the brain and analyzed. From this analyzing center a nerve impulse is sent by way of an efferent nerve to the salivary glands causing them to salivate. If at the same time, or just before the above, some other sensory nerve is stimulated, the impulses are for some reason attracted also to the salivary center in the brain. In other words, from other excited regions of the body, neural pathways are opened up to the salivary center in the brain. However, these "accidental" stimulus-response arcs are unstable and will usually disappear if not reinforced. If the accidental or conditioned pathways are strengthened through repetition, or by some strong emotion, they can become permanent.

While Pavlov's experiment may sound simple, we have learned many things from it. We now know that it is through the process of conditioning that we learn. In order to better understand how the effects of conditioning responses lead to learning, lets take a hypothetical example. Lets see how a child might learn or be conditioned to avoid a painful or dangerous situation.

Perhaps somewhere in the child's environment there is a large black stove. Not having experienced the sensation of "hot" the child has not learned that to touch hot things may be painful. If he should touch the stove and it were hot, the painful stimulus may be so severe that he is conditioned, once and for all, to avoid touching it again. On the other hand, he may try touching it several times before the avoidance response becomes conditioned.

Lets see how this can lead to situations that affect the child in later life. Suppose the child accidentally falls against the stove and is severely burned. This may so strongly condition the child he cannot be made to go near the stove again. The big black stove signals pain, and the response is avoidance. The signal may become generalized to the extent that the child avoids anything big and black. Conditioning may also occur from other signals present at the time; the color of the walls, the sound of the teakettle, even people in the room. In later life the child may have grown into an adult who feels anxious upon seeing a big black automobile. This may be true even though the incident of the burn has long since been forgotten and the fear of stoves extinguished.

An adult may dislike, or feel anxious, upon seeing a certain color or hearing a certain sound without being able to understand or explain why. Such responses are undoubtedly due to past conditioning that he can no longer recall.

Such conditioned nerve pathways are not all negative or unadaptive; fortunately most are positive or constructive and make living much easier for us. The negative ones cause such human ailments as fear, anxiety, guilt, tension and pain.

Sensory information reaching the nervous system as the result of objects that man and other animals can see or feel are the primary signals of reality. Through the process of conditioning we learn to respond to them in certain ways. The conditioned stimulus-response arcs that the primary signals trigger determine the behavior of man and animal alike.

Habits are reactions and responses that we have learned to perform automatically without having to "think" or "decide." We are conditioned to carry them out by our stimulus-response (S-R) arcs. More than 95 percent of our behavior is habitual. The typist does not "decide" which finger to put where or what key to strike. The reaction is automatic and unthinking. In much the same way our attitudes, emotions and beliefs tend to become habitual.

Most habits, can be modified, changed or reversed, simply by practicing or "acting out" the new response or behavior in our imagination. Decide what you would like to be and have, then picture yourself acting and feeling that way. Dwell upon them -- keep going over them in your mind. Generate enough emotion, or deep feeling and your new thoughts and ideas will form neural pathways. Once these new S-R arcs are formed these new ideas will be automatically carried out with out any conscious effort on your part.

An inner speech stimulus is a statement you make to yourself. The statements that we will make to ourselves in order to change our behavior are called auto-suggestions. The words you say to yourself tend to make you act in certain ways, according to your words. Your auto-suggestions can and do form S-R arcs.

Try it for yourself. Start now. Every day, several times each hour say these words to yourself over and over: "Each day I will practice the Semantic Relaxation Exercise." Remember; just say these words over and over to yourself throughout the day. Also say the words to yourself as you go to sleep tonight, and as you awaken in the morning. Then see how you are inclined to carry out this suggestion.

134

Don't assume it works, actually make the experiment. This is very important. You must get the "feel" of these methods.

S-R arcs can be conditioned by implicit kinesthetic movements. Try this: Close your eyes and then open and close your hand. What you feel is the movements of the muscles, tendons, and joints of your hand. This "muscle sense" is known as kinesthesis. It is through this sense that you know the position of your arms and legs without looking at them.

Your muscle movements are of two kinds: (1) Explicit and (2) Implicit. Your explicit movements can be seen; your implicit muscular movements cannot be seen. However, the implicit movements create a stimulus. The stimulus, in turn, brings about a S-R arc inside you.

You can easily experience the effect of your implicit muscular movements. Go where you will not be disturbed. Sit down and relax. Now close your eyes and for five minutes concentrate all your inner implicit muscle movements on the activity of writing a letter to a certain friend. Without moving, feel yourself writing the letter. Do this for five minutes. Now -- do you feel inclined to write a letter? As a matter of fact, you may actually write it. These implicit kinesthetic movements are important stimuli. They condition S-R arcs just as do visual images and verbal suggestions. The more of these mechanisms you can use at one time the more quickly and strongly will your desired responses become conditioned.

Select any act you wish to perform. Visualize everything you should see when you perform the act correctly. Learn to say the words to yourself that describe the perfect performance of the act. Learn to feel your muscles, on the implicit level, perform the act correctly. Then while you are comfortable seated, or lying down, and without appearing to move a muscle, put the three activities together. Carry out all at the same time.

We always act, feel and perform in accordance with what we imagine to be true about ourselves and our environment. We act and feel not the way things really are, but according to the image our mind holds of what they are like. We have certain mental images of ourselves, the world and people around us. We behave as though these images were true, reality, rather than the things they represent. It does not matter if these ideas and images are self-induced or come from the external world, the mental image we hold of ourselves becomes the blueprint, and our nervous system uses every means to carry out the picture. In short, we will "act like" the sort of person we conceive ourselves to be. Not only this, but we literally cannot act otherwise, in spite of all our conscious efforts or "will power." The man who conceives himself to be a "failure type person" will find some way to fail, in spite of all his good intentions. Even if opportunity is literally dumped in his lap he will not see it. The person who sees himself to be a victim injustice, one "who was meant to suffer" will invariably find circumstances to verify his opinions.

135

Many people suffer from chronic anxiety, which is simply a subconscious mental expectancy that something terrible is going to happen to them. On the other hand, we all know people who seem to have the "magic touch." Life seems to shower them with blessings for no apparent reason. We call them "lucky." What seems to be luck is in reality, POSITIVE MENTAL EXPECTANCY, a strong belief that they deserve to be successful.

Our physical health is largely dependent upon our mental expectancy. Physicians recognize that if a patient expects to remain sick, lame, paralyzed or helpless, the expected condition tends to be realized. Self-hypnosis and autosuggestion can become the tools with which to remove negative attitudes and replace them with positive expectancy.

Once an idea has been accepted, it tends to remain. The longer it is held, the more it tends to become a fixed habit of thinking. This is how habits are formed, both good and bad. First there is the thought and then the action. We have habits of thinking as well as habits of action, but the thought or idea always comes first. Therefore, if we wish to change our actions we must begin by changing our thoughts. We accept as true certain facts. For example, we accept as true that the sun rises in the east and sets in the west. We accept this even though the day may be cloudy and we cannot see the sun. This is an instance of a correct fact conception that governs our actions under normal conditions. However, we have many thought habits that are not correct and are fixed in the mind. Some people believe that at critical times they must have a drink of whisky or a tranquilizer to steady their nerves so that they can perform effectively. This is not correct, but the idea is there, and is a fixed habit of thought. We need to alter ideas or use them. No matter how fixed the ideas may be or how long they have remained, they can be changed with self-hypnosis and autosuggestion.

There is an abundance of experimental evidence demonstrating that thinking is accomplished by muscular contractions. These are so slight that they can only be detected by sensitive electronic instruments. It has been demonstrated (Totten, 1935) that a person thinking of a geometric design will move his eyes to correspond with the outline of it. Of all the indications of emotion, the most easily measured are the visceral changes that take place throughout the body. The external responses to anger may be consciously controlled by an individual; his visceral responses however are not subject to voluntary control. If you could look directly into his blood stream you would find an excessive amount of adrenaline present. His liver would have released stored sugar into the blood. Chemical changes would have occurred in the blood causing it to clot more quickly. The blood pressure will have risen and the heart will beat more rapidly and vigorously. The air passages into the lungs will have enlarged. The pupils of the eyes will have enlarged. Sweat will have broken out all over the body, particularly on the palms of the hands. The temperature of the skin may have risen or fallen several degrees.

Other emotions will cause different visceral changes in the body. Sorrow will cause the actions of the heart and lungs to decrease while that of the gallbladder will increase. Fear will cause the activity of the stomach to stop. The adrenal glands become very active. During feelings of joy the whole body functions well, with the stomach very active.

Ideas that have a strong emotional content almost always tend to form S-R arcs. Once these arcs are formed, the ideas will continue to produce the same physical reactions over and over again. In order to eliminate chronic negative ideas that cause harmful physical reactions, we must replace them with positive ones. This is easily done with self-hypnosis and autosuggestion.

Stress and tension may serve to lower the body's natural resistance to infectious diseases and in this sense it could be said that all illness has an emotional background. Some of the more common bodily ailments which result from sustained emotional tensions are: alcoholism, most allergies, asthma, bronchitis, Buerger's disease, common cold, constipation, colitis, coronary heart disease, diarrhea, drug addiction, diabetes mellitus, emphysema, eczema, enuresis (bed wetting), epilepsy (some forms), frigidity, gallbladder disease, goiter, hives, hay fever, hemorrhoids, high blood pressure, hiccups, hyperthyroidism, hypoglycemia, habitual abortion, infertility, impotence, migraine, multiple sclerosis, myasthenia gravis, obesity, premature ejaculation, paroxysmal tachycardia (sudden rapid heart beat), Reynauld's disease, sinusitis, tic douloureux, trigeminal neuralgia, and urticaria.

PSYCHOSOMATIC DISORDERS

Many illnesses have for some time been recognized as "nervous" or functional disorders. That is, disorders for which there is no known organic bases. Many of you have probably experienced "nervous headaches." The relationship of insomnia to worry is well known. What is perhaps not so well known is that worry is one of the greatest causes of illness and fatigue. Some people have chronic illnesses or have loved ones that are ill or away at war. We can hardly expect such people to stop worrying. However, there are many people that have developed a habit of worrying. They constantly worry over needless or foolish things, and as a result make themselves sick. Many people worry about something every day of their lives. If they can't find something real to worry about they will usually make up something.

A wealthy woman of 55 with an affectionate family, a beautiful home and perfect health worried herself sick. She felt since good fortune had smiled on her all her life, it was about time some disaster befell her or one of her loved ones. As a result, every time the telephone rang she went all to pieces for fear it would bring news of some disaster that had overtaken her husband or one of her children.

I have seen hundreds of very unhappy people who feel because of bad judgment on their part; they have contributed to the illness or death of a parent, husband or wife. They keep saying over and over, "If I had only called another physician, or refused to permit the operation, the disaster would not have happened." They do not seem to realize that the Good Lord only expects us to do the very best we can. He does not expect us to have the ability to look into the future.

Many people will worry for years over some problem that could be solved in a few minutes by their physician, lawyer or banker. People can and do literally worry themselves to death over nothing. Such chronic worrying is a conditioned response that can easily be changed with self-hypnosis and autosuggestion.

Many psychosomatic disorders are well known. Some of you may know people who at some time or another have suffered from psychogenic varieties of diarrhea, asthma, hives, constipation, hay fever, peptic ulcer, or high blood pressure. The list is long and growing day by day. Less generally appreciated is the manner in which mental activity can influence the course of an organic disease such as tuberculosis or cancer. Well known, but less understood is a wide class of diseases known as hysteria. A person suffering from this disorder can become suddenly blind, paralyzed, or deaf. As suddenly as the symptom may disappear only to be replaced by another hysterical symptom.

It is through the autonomic nervous system (ANS) that the physical dysfunctions are initiated and aggravated by our mental activity. In order to better understand how this comes about we will take a closer look at some of the specific functions of the two branches of the ANS and at the phenomenon of parasympathetic overcompensation.

If we were to examine each psychosomatic disorder individually we would fine the ANS involved in each of them. The following three examples are presented in order that you may gain some understanding of how the ANS is involved in psychosomatic disorders. The three examples are: (1) Activity of the sweat glands, which are enervated solely by the sympathetic branch. (2) The secretion of hydrochloric acid in the stomach, which is under the control of the parasympathetic branch. (3) The mucous membrane lining of the lungs, which is under the control of both branches of the ANS.

It is very well known that sweat changes are very reliable indicators of ANS activity and can readably be measured and recorded electronically. Some individuals due to past conditioning have extremely reactive sweat glands. Even in the resting state the electrical resistance of their palms is low and with any emotional situation which activates the sympathetic nervous system (SNS), it drops even lower as they sweat more profusely from their palms and soles of their feet, armpits and some facial areas. Sweating from the hands is particularly noticeable. If such a person should fine himself in an intense emotional situation he sweats so profusely from his hands that it becomes intolerable to him. The beads of perspiration appear almost immediately at the onset of any emotional situation that affects the SNS, and will remain as long as the emotional tension lasts. Such an individual may only have dry hands while asleep.

This condition of hyperhydrolsis is typical in many individuals that are hyper-emotional. Such a condition may be helped by drugs or surgically by cutting the nerves that supply such areas. However, this will not change other SNS activity that accompanies such a condition. Nor will it greatly alter the emotional reactivity of the individual. The ideal way to correct such a situation is to change the conditioned emotional response. This can be accomplished through relearning. Then, and only then, will total SNS activity be reduced. Such relearning of emotional responses can be greatly facilitated through hypnosis.

Our second example, the secreting of hydrochloric acid, was selected because it is one of the few functions of the body that is solely under the control of the parasympathetic nervous system (PNS). Alone it is of little interest, together with other functions inebriated by the PNS it is of tremendous importance. In certain emotional situations there can be an excessive amount of hydrochloric acid secreted. Generally this excessive secretion of hydrochloric acid is accompanied by increases in other PNS activity. There is often hyperactivity of the stomach and an increase in the amount of blood supplied to the viscera. In some cases there is a decrease in the mucous lining of the stomach. Lets combine these events and see what happens.

Typically during fear or anxiety the above conditions are inhibited. The secretion of hydrochloric acid is decreased, less blood is supplied to the stomach wall and the stomach becomes less active. However, during some emotions, such as chronic resentment, the situation may be reversed. There is an excessive secretion of hydrochloric acid, an increase in stomach activity and blood supply. Minute hemorrhages may occur in the walls of the stomach. If there is a decrease in the mucous lining of the stomach during such a state, we have an ideal situation for the production of ulcers. There is a rich blood supply to an over active stomach which, with or without minute hemorrhages, becomes more sensitive to the action of hydrochloric acid. Under such conditions hydrochloric acid begins to consume the lining of the stomach and an ulcer is born. While it is known that emotions, such as resentment, can directly trigger the PNS, more profound emotions seem to be followed by over PNS activity after some time has elapsed. It is suspected that initial SNS activity is sometimes followed by a period of increased PNS activity which is regarded as over compensatory in nature. However, more research is needed before this phenomenon can be understood. It is certain though; the events leading to the development of a stomach or intestinal ulcer are the result of over activity on the part of the PNS. As with the case of hyperhydrosis, the symptoms can be treated by drugs or surgery. But again, re-education is the method of choice. By learning new conditioned responses not only will the ulcer-tendency be reduced, but also the tendency to develop other psychosomatic disorders. Again, hypnosis is probably the quickest and least expensive method available today.

Among the psychosomatic diseases we listed was asthma. The asthmatic tends to have great difficulty breathing at times. Sometimes he is described as allergic to pollen or other substances. Sometimes no evidence of allergy can be found. Always there is excessive enervation of the PNS leading to the lungs. The mucus cells are forced to over secrete and the blood vessels supplying the lungs are dilated accompanied by swelling of tissues. In other words, the air passages become congested and breathing becomes difficult. The classic method of treating acute cases is an injection of adrenalin. Adrenalin acts a powerful stimulant on the SNS. A dramatic change takes place. The mucous secretion stops, the blood vessels and the tissue around them constrict. The individual can then breath. Anyone that has ever used a "benzedrine inhaler" has experienced the same thing in the mucous tissues of the nose.

In the above case, surgery is ruled out as the branches of the vagus nerves that enervate the lungs are easily confused with those supplying the heart. Again, the most effective therapy is re-education. The individual can be reconditioned so that his PNS will no longer over react to stressful situations.

139

MUSCULAR TENSION

Muscular tension plays a large part in our emotional states and psychosomatic conditions. Smooth muscle, the type of muscle found in the organs of the body is under the control of the ANS. These muscles are generally not considered to be under voluntary control. These muscles are in a state of more or less constant activity. Their general pattern of activity is one of slow increase or decrease of muscular tone.

It is possible for skeletal, or voluntary muscles, of the body to maintain various states of tension. This is typical of the antigravity muscles (those muscles that help us maintain our posture). They are called antigravity muscles because they oppose the force of gravity when one is in an upright position. During most of our waking hours, some or all of these muscles are in a state of tension. However, there is a marked difference between individuals.

We are all familiar with the person that is tense most of the time. His movements seen to be jerky, his face expressive and sometimes contorted. He rarely seems to relax and take things easy. Not quite as often we see the opposite extreme. He is the individual who seems so relaxed he gives the impression of being almost asleep. His arms swing freely and loosely from his shoulders. His movements are often rather lethargic, his facial muscles seem to hang loose or to be sagging. He seldom, if ever, goes into quick action. Most of us lie somewhere in between the two extremes, and some of us are capable of optimum differential relaxation.

Differential relaxation is a condition that is worth considerable effort to learn. In some individuals it seems to occur naturally. That is, without any conscious effort or learning. In many others however, it does not seem to occur naturally, and a great deal of practice is necessary in order to achieve it. That it can be achieved has been demonstrated by anyone who has studied yoga.

The lack of differential muscular reaction is obvious in the act of writing. Tension in certain muscle groups is necessary for the act of writing. We must exert enough tension to hold the pen or pencil we are using. Tension is involved in the upper arm muscles in order to move the hand that contains the writing instrument. Of course, the antigravity muscles must maintain a degree of tension to keep us in an upright position.

Most of us go beyond this necessary minimum amount of muscular tension. While it is only necessary to maintain a tight grip on the pencil while writing, most of us continue the pressure between words or while thinking what to write next. Sometimes we start the grip before we actually start writing. Often we maintain it once we have completed a sentence for a long time.

This lack of differential relaxation is not confined to the hand and arm muscles. The person that does not relax between actual writing will probably not be relaxed in other portions of his body. He is apt to be sitting on the edge of his chair. He is often observed to be engaged in restless movements with the legs, the feet, the unoccupied hand, and the head and neck muscles. In other words, he is tense throughout his body. Usually such individuals find it difficult to relax when they retire. They often complain of difficulty in falling asleep or of tenseness in various parts of their body.

The most important fact we wish to emphasize is that whenever we experience profound emotion, tension in the skeletal muscles also increases. Whenever you become angry or frightened, not only is your ANS activated but your skeletal muscles as well. The increase of muscular tension in turn facilitates the emotional experience. In general, as our emotional state increases, our muscles become more tense, but also, with increased muscle tension we become more emotional. Therefore, any factor that will increase muscular tension will also increase emotional behavior and other psychosomatic functions. This is why some psychotherapists (including the Yogis) concentrate upon techniques for inducing muscular relaxation. How often have you told a friend, "Just relax, everything will be alright?" Muscular tension and relaxation are important in human behavior. Any factor that will decrease tension in skeletal muscles will alleviate psychosomatic problems.

As many experiments have shown, practically any function of the body can be conditioned to practically any stimulus. Muscular tension is no exception. We have mentioned the tendency of some people to grasp a pencil firmly before they even start to write. In other words they are "set" to begin to write. The word "set" is commonly used for the runner. For him the signals "On your mark" and "get set" have a different meaning. He has learned through practice the most efficient kinds of neuro-muscular responses to such stimuli. They are conditioned muscular tension patterns. The first are less intense, less intensive. The second are more intense and extensive.

The term "get set" is used under all kinds of situations. We are set to throw, we are set to run, or we are set to talk. You can picture yourself in anyone of these situations and actually set yourself for each of these reactions. In each case you will realize that there are changes in the tone of the various striate muscles throughout your body. Each of these changes represent a conditioned response to different stimuli and each prepares you for a definite type of activity that you have learned. In fact, when we say we are set for a specific activity, we are implying that we have learned that act, and that we have learned a preparatory muscular tension pattern that is effective in carrying out that act. Through conditioning (a form of learning) we say we may get "set" to carry out many types of reactions -- for running, for walking, for listening, for sweating, for ulcers or for asthma.

RULES OF THE MIND

RULE I

WHAT IS IMAGINED OR EXPECTED TENDS TO BE REALIZED

Dr. Maxwell Maltz, in his popular book "Psycho-Cybernetics," describes the subconscious mind as a "goal-striving mechanism." This term means that when the mind perceives a goal it automatically works to achieve that goal.

The individual, who strongly believes in success, subconsciously strives to bring about favorable circumstances leading to success. When advantageous conditions arise, he is able to recognize the opportunity and take the steps necessary to complete his success plan. We all know people who seem to have a "magic touch." Life seems to shower them with blessings for no apparent reason and we call them "lucky." What appears to be luck is actually nothing more than POSITIVE MENTAL EXPECTANCY -- a strong belief and mental image of success.

On the other hand, the person who conceives himself to be a "failure type" will find some way to fail, in spite of all good intentions. The student who believes he is poor in arithmetic must make poor grades in that subject to justify his own convictions. His original negative belief is reaffirmed by his poor grades and a vicious cycle is set in motion.

Expect good things to happen and good things will occur. Vividly imagine yourself successful and you will achieve success.

RULE II

EVERY THOUGHT OR IDEA PRODUCES A PHYSICAL RESPONSE

An abundance of experimental data on thought processes has revealed that thinking is always accomplished by some physical response. Many scientists believe that muscular movements are an integral part of the thought process. For example, whenever we think of a word, our vocal muscles react and become part of the thought. To convince yourself of this phenomenon, try the following exercise: Holding your mouth wide open, try to think the word "bubble." Upon first trying this you may find it very difficult to think the word, or the thought may at first seem slurred, as though you were attempting to pronounce the word aloud with your mouth held open.

Thoughts and ideas with strong emotional content produce physical responses in the body characteristic of the emotion. Anger and fear thoughts stimulate the adrenal glands that in turn affect the activity of most body functions. Recent studies have shown that the body's natural resistance to disease can even be affected by one's thoughts and emotions.

In order to adapt successfully to the stresses of life and eliminate or change chronic negative physical reactions, we must first learn to change our THINKING HABITS. We must learn to accept

142

situations positively. We must learn to change fixed negative ideas into strong positive attitudes. This can be done with autosuggestion and self-hypnosis.

RULE III

LAW OF REVERSED EFFECT

This law was first formulated around the turn of the century. Emile Coue, the father of autosuggestion referred to it as the "Law of Reversed Effort." Coue stated, "whenever there is a conflict between the will (conscious effort) and the imagination (mental imagery), not only do we not do that which we wish, but we do the exact opposite." When one thinks that he would like to do something but feels he cannot, then the more he tries the more difficult it becomes.

A common example of this rule is seen in people troubled with insomnia. They go to bed with the thought "I suppose I'll not be able to sleep." Then they try and the harder they try the more wide-awake they become. Sometime later, thoroughly fatigued, they stop trying; begin to think of something else and drop off to sleep within a few minutes.

A second example of the Law of Reversed Effect is the forgetting of a name. The more you consciously try to remember the forgotten name the more impossible it becomes. Later, when you have stopped trying and are thinking of something else, the name easily comes to mind.

The attitude reflected in the Law of Reversed Effect is: I want very much to do it, but I know that I cannot. What is expected then tends to be realized (Rule I) and you obtain the opposite of that which you seek.

RULE IV

NEW HABIT PATTERNS CAN BE FORMED WITH VISUALIZED IMAGES

When you look at an object, light reflected from the object enters your eyes causing an electrochemical change to occur. This changes produces nerve impulses that are transmitted to the visual center of your brain where they are interpreted as visual images. It is these mental images in the brain that you react to and not the actual object itself. For this reason, visualizing some object or action in your imagination can have the same affect as the real event.

143

Realizing that our nervous system cannot tell the difference between an actual experience and one that is vividly imagined opens a new door to self-improvement. It offers the opportunity to practice, without effort, new skills, traits and attitudes until new habit patterns are formed. Habit patterns can be modified and even reversed simply by practicing or "acting out" the new response or behavior in your imagination. However, this rule can work for or against you. An imagination preoccupied with negative images will only serve to hinder your improvement.

Successful living starts with a picture held in your imagination -- a picture of what you want to be and of what you want to accomplish. Decide how you want to act, then picture yourself acting and feeling that way. Dwell upon those ideas -- keep going over them in your mind and new habit patterns will begin to form. Once the habit patterns are established, the desired result will occur automatically without conscious effort.

RULE V

HABIT PATTERNS CAN BE FORMED WITH AUTO-SUGGESTIONS

Words, whether spoken or unspoken, are symbols that convey certain images and thoughts to the mind through previous associations. When we think the word "HOT," for example, an image immediately comes to mind relating to some experience of being hot, of being burned by something hot, or of a hot object. Once a word becomes associated with a specific image (object or action), the word alone then becomes a signal to the mind representative of that image and can act to elicit the same responses that the image itself would evoke.

Kimball Young once said, "words are an expansion and creation of total reality." Through the use of words, in the form of autosuggestions, we are able to create "real" situations corresponding to the goals we seek to achieve. Repetitious use of autosuggestions then act to form new patterns of behavior.

Because repeated use of words and thoughts can act to form new habit patterns, we must be careful in our everyday life to repeat words and thoughts that result in productive responses and avoid negative words and thoughts that evoke destructive responses. It is also important to realize that when someone else says something it becomes your thought for the moment. Therefore it is equally important to avoid situations in which you are continually exposed to negative words, negative thoughts, and negative goals.

You will be given specific rules for structuring positive autosuggestions (see Rules for Structuring Autosuggestions) and you will learn how to effectively administer these suggestions in a scientific manner (see Rules for Administering Autosuggestions).

RULE VI

ATTITUDES AND HABITS ARE BEST LEARNED OR CHANGED WITHOUT EFFORT

Out currently held beliefs, whether good or bad, true or false, were formed without effort, with no sense of strain, and without the exercise of "will power." Habit patterns whether good or bad are formed in the same way.

The late Dr. Knight Dunlap made a life long study of habits and learning processes. His findings revealed that effort was the one big deterrent to either breaking a bad habit or forming a new one. In many cases, effort to change an undesirable habit may actually serve to reinforce the habit. His studies proved that the best way to break a bad habit is to form a clear mental image of the desired end result, and to practice without effort toward reaching that goal.

Instead of trying hard by conscious effort and "iron-jaw" will power to change undesirable habits, simply let yourself relax, mentally picture yourself as you want to be and allow the new habit patterns to form automatically. Once the new habit pattern has started, it will automatically strengthen itself with each repetition and each successful performance.

RULE VII

ONCE A HABIT PATTERN HAS BEEN ESTABLISHED, IT TENDS TO REMAIN UNTIL REPLACED WITH A NEW PATTERN OF BEHAVIOR

Starting at birth, and from then on, every individual is continually exposed to a variety of situations requiring some degree of adaptive behavior. Similar situations occurring repeatedly soon begin to establish certain conditioned responses. Once this happens, each repeated occurrence serves to reinforce the responses, until they become so strongly established that we are unable to exercise much voluntary control over them. If all habits, attitudes and emotions were beneficial there would be no problems. Unfortunately, often they are not.

To change a habit pattern, we begin by forming new conditioned response patterns for the habit situation. We then practice the new responses, using techniques found here (Self-Hypnosis Center's Home Page), until they become so strongly associated with the habit situation that a new pattern of behavior is formed. A person with stage fright, for example, can easily learn to associate feeling of

145

confidence, poise and success with situations requiring his performance in front of an audience. As the new response pattern becomes stronger with each repetition, the old responses are permanently replaced.

RULE VIII

HABIT PATTERNS CAN BE FORMED WITHOUT REPETITION

Many reflexes are present at birth and others are acquired through repeated experiences. However, reflexes and behavior patterns can be formed from a single experience. When any strong emotion is present there is an intense focusing of mental activity and undesirable reflex responses may develop accidentally. For example, a child who is barked at, chased or bitten by a dog rapidly learns to fear dogs. Only one such encounter may cause the child to subsequently fear all dogs, even harmless pictures of dogs.

A similar condition of focused mental activity can be brought about intentionally to form desirable behavior patterns with little or no repetition. The process occurs most easily when the body is completely relaxed and all competing or conflicting thoughts and ideas are held to a minimum. Carefully structured auto-suggestions and mental imagery can be used during this time to rapidly develop new habit patterns.

LANGUAGE

There are many similarities between man and the lower animals. They are both capable of learning to various degrees. It has been demonstrated that some animals are able to reason to some extant. For example, if food is placed outside the reach of a caged monkey that has been provided with sticks when joined together will reach the food, the monkey will soon join the sticks and retrieve the food. This is possible because of the monkey's ability to think creatively. Man and animal learn in the same way; through sensory information reaching the nervous system as a result of objects and events that can be seen or felt. Through a process called conditioning (classical or operant) all animals learn to respond to these objects and events in certain ways. The way we learn to respond to these objects and events in the real world outside of our skin determines the behavior of animal and man alike.

There is however one great difference between the human animal and all other animals. This one factor has made it possible for man to rise supreme over all other animals on this planet. This single factor is his ability to use WORDS. The invention of speech is man's greatest discovery. The importance of semantic or articulated language cannot be over emphasized.

There are many books and classes dealing with self-help available, but in all systems, the most important factor is overlooked. The language we use! We depend on language for thoughts, for ideas, and for the most part we think in words. Yet we tend to overlook their influence on us.

While it is possible to think without using words, this type of thinking is very limited and very primitive. Although we can only guess what an animal experiences, it is probable that a hungry dog has a mental image of the meat he would like to eat. In this sense he is "thinking" about the piece of meat. But he does not have a symbol (word) for meat, or for the general category food. Man does not require words to decide how to dress himself in the morning. A series of mental pictures is sufficient for this purpose. But thinking without the aid of verbal symbols is limited to the simplest of matters.

We need words to deal with abstract ideas -- ideas such as "justice", "happiness" and "success," which unlike such words as "chair", "ball" and "dog" stand for entities that cannot be seen or touched.

Words are symbols that stand for objects, actions or ideas. For example, the word "table" is a symbol that stands for that article of furniture we sometimes eat from. The advantages of a thinking system bases on symbols or words are tremendous. We do not have to see a table to deal with it mentally. The word "table" stands for all the characteristics and functions we observe in that article of furniture. Once it is tagged with a name, we know without studying a table what it has in common with other objects like it. Words therefore shorten and streamline the learning process.

As great as this system of human thought may be, if we are not very careful there can be serious and disastrous disadvantages. As we have learned to react to objects and events in the real world at a subconscious level, so we learn to respond to words at a subconscious level. The difficulty is this: We tend to respond to words as though they were what they symbolized. However, words are not the things they stand for. For example, the word "steak" cannot be eaten. The word "chair" cannot be sat upon. On first hearing this most people respond by thinking, "That's obvious, everyone knows that." However, it is not as apparent as you think.

Let us give you a simple example to illustrate how we subconsciously respond to words as though they were what they represent. If the word "fire" were shouted when you were sitting in a crowded theater your reaction would most likely be instantaneous -- a panic response. You would experience fear; you may tremble and feel your heart pounding violently. Your mouth may feel dry. You may experience a sensation of hollowness in your stomach. Your blood pressure will either fall or rise.

Your face may turn white. Your legs and arms may feel week and helpless. In this paralysis of fear, action may be impossible.

Now stop and think. To what did your body react to with such profound changes? Your entire body responded to a single word. The word "fire." You did not see any flames. You did not smell any smoke. You did not feel any pain. You did not feel the warmth of the fire. Your reaction was to a word.

Because there is a symbol or word called "bad," many people make the subconscious assumption there is something that exists in the real world called "badness." It does not. "Badness" cannot be tasted, touched, weighted or measured, it is an abstract concept.

Man is the only animal that makes war on members of his own species in the name of such abstract concepts as "justice" and "patriotism," or in the defense of political and economic philosophies. The ape and lion will fight ferociously to defend their property rights, but only if his territory is in immediate danger of attack. On the other hand, one needs WORDS to convince people who live half a world away to fight for a territory they cannot see and with which they are not directly concerned. Only through language can man be convinced to leave his home and family in order to defend, not the mountains, plains and waterways of his country, but the principles for which that country stands.

Very few of us are aware of the degree to which we are controlled by the words we use and hear. We become conditioned to respond in set ways to some words so that our responses to them are completely predictable. Mr. Jones will never vote for a "democrat" no matter how untrustworthy the other candidates may be. Mr. Smith always disapproves of strikes and strikers, without bothering to find out if a particular strike is justified or not. Mr. Thompson sympathizes with all strikers because he hates all bosses.

Our prejudices are fixed reactions that are triggered by words we have been conditioned to respond to in set ways. Mr. Smith fears and distrusts all people that are called "Catholics." Mr. Jones is a Catholic; he fears and distrusts all non-Catholics. Mr. Wilson is such a rabid republican that when L. B. Johnson was president, he not only disliked the Democratic President but also his wife, children and dogs. Mr. Miller, a rabid democrat, gave up golf during the Eisenhower administration (he resumed it after Kennedy took up the game). Such people treat all democrats, republicans, bosses, and strikers as if they were all the same -- they are not. As well as seeing the similarities between things it is also important to realize that there are differences and that no two thing are ever exactly alike. Ham and eggs (Ritz Hotel) are not ham and eggs (Joe's Bar and Grill). Private enterprise (Bill's Garage) is not private enterprise (General Motors). Wendell Johnson summed it up when he said. "To a mouse, cheese is cheese -- that's why mousetraps work."

148

Words have meaning far beyond the meanings given to them in the most extensive dictionary. Therefore, they have no "general meaning," in spite of the dictionary. We are interested in words as they affect us subconsciously; affect our nervous system and our entire body.

When you are not feeling too well, or when you think you might be ill, you are apt to say to yourself, "I am sick." Simple words, aren't they? However, their power can drive people into the depth of despair and disease. As soon as you say, "I am sick," your nervous system relays the message to your entire body, which responds with a letdown. This letdown may first be felt as a lethargy or depression, and if you feel this way, you can imagine what is happening to the cells and organs of your body. They too get depressed. That is, their normal function is interfered with, and when this happens, the individual is on the road to true illness or a more serious ailment than he or she ought to have. What you believe, what you think, more than you realize, actually is so -- or soon can be. Our own words can make us well or sick, a failure or a success. What is the difference between the man that has failed in business three times and says, "I am a failure," and the man that says, "I have failed three times?" The difference is that between self-destruction and sanity.

THE POWER OF YOUR CREATIVE IMAGINATION

It is being realized more and more by big corporations, as well as by individuals, the value of a fertile imagination. It is the fountain of all creative thinking. Most men and women in the higher salary brackets are there not because of hard work, but because they have active creative imaginations. One of the primary reasons most people are unsuccessful is because they have never learned to use their imagination. We are all born with very active imaginations. Every child has a very active imagination. In fact most children live in a fantasy world for a number of years. It is a normal phase of personality development. However, as the higher reasoning powers begin to rapidly mature, the child progresses into a world of realism. This is a critical development period as far as the imagination is concerned. Many young people almost completely quit using their imagination at this phase of their lives. Others (i.e., those interested in the arts) begin to make use of their imagination in a constructive way. Parents play an important role at this point. Some will give their children some creative outlet for their imagination; others will stifle or inhibit the child's imagination.

Often the imagination flourishes during the later adolescent years until the individual has a collision with the hard cruel world of adult reality. When this happens, many young people cease using their imagination. If they have been hurt and disillusioned by the realities of the world, they feel if they allow their imagination to function it will create new experiences where they are hurt and discouraged. At least this is what they subconsciously tell themselves.

In reality, every human being has an imagination. It may be repressed, inactive, or distorted, but it exists. When many people are asked if they have a good imagination. Most will reply that they have no imagination (40 to 50 percent). Others claim they have too much imagination; they lost their imagination years ago, or ask, "what do you mean by imagination?" The important question is not if you have an imagination (you do), but what are you doing with it?

149

If we were to ask you, "What is more powerful, your imagination or your will-power?" what would your answer be? The reality is, your imagination is far more powerful than your will-power. Emile Coue answered this question during the last century (See Rules of the Mind). He demonstrated that when there is a conflict between the imagination and will-power, the imagination wins every time. You can use your will-power all you want to keep on a slimming diet, but when you begin to imagine how good that dessert tastes, all your iron-jawed will-power will not help you.

All the great concepts and inventions of mankind were born in the imagination. Before Beethoven, Bach or any of the great composers wrote a musical composition, they first heard the music in their mind. Rembrandt saw his painting in his imagination before he put them on canvas. Every architect sees his creations in his head before he puts them on the drawing board. Every great writer writes his stories in his imagination before putting them on paper. How can you be a successful inventor without an active imagination? First, in your mind you must see a need for your invention. You must then visualize a way to fulfill that need. Then you must design the product in your imagination before actually creating it.

The constructive use of the imagination is important to everyone. No matter if you are an artist, engineer, physicist, or businessman, the way you use your imagination will determine the future course of your life. America is still a land where a man can begin with nothing but an idea and turn it into multimillion-dollar corporation.

If you do not use your imagination constructively, it can inhibit you and work against you. If you imagine that something you want to do is too difficult you may not even try to start a project. Most difficulties that people face in life exist more often in their imaginations than in actual fact. These negative thoughts created in your imagination generate fear, and if it is great enough, it will prevent you from even trying to achieve anything.

The improper use of you imagination can undermine you. Probably every one is familiar with the proverbial daydreamer. This is the individual that is always building "pie in the sky." In reality he never produces anything. He spends his time waiting for his ship to come in, but it never does. When your imagination prevents you from engaging in productive activity, it is being misused. People that sit around fantasizing and daydreaming, but who accomplish nothing, are not creative thinkers.

Individuals with creative imaginations produce! Their goals are realistic. Alexander Graham Bell didn't just fantasize about talking to someone over a great distance. He used his imagination to create an instrument to make it possible -- he invented the telephone. Today we can talk to anyone anywhere in the world thanks to his creative imagination. The light bulb was born in Thomas Edison's imagination. In his day there were no light bulbs, except in his mind. He believed it was a practical idea and set about to prove it. Can a man fly? They could in the imaginations of a couple of brothers named Orville and Wilbur Wright. They proved it at a desolate place called Kitty Hawk on December 17, 1903.

You have to make a distinction between idle daydreaming and creative, productive thinking. The former can destroy you, and the latter can lead you to a happy successful life. Daydreaming is just a form of procrastination; it is a misuse of your imagination that will get you nowhere.

If you use your imagination in a positive, constructive way, you can improve all aspects of your daily life. People tend to create mental pictures of everyone they know. The image is base on the knowledge you have about your acquaintances, and associations you make with them and other people you have known. You seldom see them as an individual, but as a composite of others that fit into a certain image category. Your imagination plays a large role in how you feel about an individual therefore it plays a major role in your human relationships.

Your imagination, when used wisely, can be a valuable tool in helping you realize your full potential in life. It can play a vital part in increasing your income, your self-confidence, improving your human relationships, school grades, and your creative abilities. You will discover abilities and talents you didn't know you had.

Here are some pointers on how you can immediately begin to increase the power of your creative imagination:

"   You should recognize and understand the power of your imagination. If you don't fully understand this fact, you will never realize your full potential in life.

"   Learn to control your imagination. Take a few minutes each day to practice seeing visual images in your mind.

"   Form a habit of always using your imagination as a preparation for constructive activity. Avoid using it for idle daydreaming. Learn to control and direct it in constructive channels.

"   Develop the creative dimension of your imagination. Visualize new products and concepts that would benefit mankind. Think of new ways to approach old problems.

"   When you have your back against the wall, let your imagination run wild. This technique is called "brain-storming." Wild thoughts often produce new solutions to difficult problems.

"   Keep practicing these techniques until you can effectively use your imagination to your benefit.

REMEMBER THESE IMPORTANT IDEAS:

1. The real secret of success is a creative imagination.

2. Everyone was born with a good imagination. You still have one, even though it may be dormant and inactive.

3. The imagination is more powerful than "will power."

4. All great accomplishments were born in the imagination.

5. Your imagination, if misused, can undermine your accomplishments.

6. You must distinguish between idle daydreaming and constructively using your imagination. A creative imagination is always constructive.

7. Your imagination can help you increase your income and improve your relationships with others.

8. Your imagination can be a big help in developing your self-hypnosis skills.

9. The sub-conscious is very responsive to your imagination.

10. Your imagination and self-hypnosis can work together to help you realize your goals.

HOW TO SET REALISTIC GOALS

In order to achieve a goal you must first have a goal. Many people really have no goals in life; they just seem to drift along with the tide. Their lives lack direction and as a result, they don't achieve much. People that know them often recognize that they are very capable people and lament the tragedy that they are not more goal directed and more successful. At the other extreme are people who constantly set their goals so very high that it is impossible to achieve them. Such people are chronically tense and miserable, because they are continually failing. Every unrealized goal is a failure. Even if they should achieve a goal, they feel it took longer than they had planed, and is therefore another failure. Such people are unable to relax, they constantly drive themselves. They may accomplish a great deal, but they never enjoy it. The fact that they were unable to achieve as much as soon as they wanted prevents them from enjoying their achievements. They become old before their time, their energy and vitality sapped by tension and anxiety. Their disillusionment turns to cynicism and depression.

Both of the above types suffer from the same basic problem. They are both unable to set realistic goals to guide them through life. Quite often the person who drifts with the tide sets very low goals or no goals at all. Usually this is due to the fear of failure. He has learned that failure causes him to become anxious and depressed. If he does not set any goals, he can't fail. However, both types end up in defeat.

In addition to setting goals that are too high or too low, you can set goals that are so vaguely formulated that you have no way of knowing if you have achieved your goal or not. Since such people are unable to really define their goals and are therefore unable to recognize them even if they should reach them, they automatically assume they have failed. Such a person may decide that his goal in life is to become successful. He expends all his energy and time trying to achieve "success." Ask him to define success and he can only give you a vague idea of what it is, but he "knows" that when he finds it he will recognize it. Success is just a word that symbolizes an abstract concept; there is no such thing as success in the real world, yet this is the one thing he wants -- success. Since it does not exist he can only fail. All anyone can hope to achieve is a series of relative successes and not some mysterious thing called success.

Your task, if you have not already done so, is to set good, realistic goals for yourself. They give direction to your life; give you a feeling of accomplishment and success as you achieve them.

In order to understand the process of setting realistic goals, you need to realize that there are LONG-TERM and SHORT-TERM goals. Long-term goals refer to major things we wish to accomplish eventually in our lives. Short-term goals refer to things we must do more or less immediately. Long-term goals are generally achieved by accomplishing many short-term goals. For example, say a person wants to become a chemist. This is a long-term goal. In order to achieve this long-term goal many short-term goals, such as, entering college, selecting the proper courses, passing tests, completing assignments, accumulating a sufficient number of credit hours, obtaining a college degree, and finding employment must be accomplished.

The Following Rules Will Help You Set Good Long-Term Goals

"   Decide if the goal is an appropriate one for you. Watch out for goals that are too high, too low or too vague. It helps to talk to others and learn from their experiences. Get advice from friends and/or professionals about whether this is a good, realistic goal for you. However, in the end, you will have to make the decision.

"   Make your long-term goals general rather than specific. If they are too specific you are inviting failure. If they are more general they can be achieved in a number of different ways. For example, it is better to set a goal of being a good contributor to the welfare of the community than deciding to be voted the most outstanding citizen by some organization and being elected the youngest mayor the city has ever had. Goals that are too specific almost end in frustration and lead to feeling of failure.

"   Once a long-term goal has been selected, analyze it in terms of the short-term goals that must be achieved to get there. Determine what path your short-term goals should take. There is almost always more than one way to achieve a long-term goal. You don't have to do it the way someone else did. Go about it in the way that it is most likely to succeed for you.

"   Start NOW! Begin working systematically on the short-term goals. Set up a time schedule that is realistic. Remember, things that are worthwhile take time. Most people underestimate the length of time it will take to accomplish a goal. Be patient with your goals, otherwise you set yourself up for frustration, tension and anxiety.

The Following Rules Will Help You Set Good Short-Term Goals

"   As with long-term goals, they should be realistic. They should be small, discrete steps leading toward the long-term goal. They should be things you can do more or less immediately.

"   They should be more specific than long-term goals. They should be specific enough to allow you to determine what you need to achieve next and where you are going.

"   Your approach to accomplishing these short-term goals should be organized and planed in such a way that you have a high probability of getting them done.

"   If you fail at one of your short-term goals, do not magnify it out of proportion. One failure or mistake does not mean that you will never reach your ultimate destination. If you should fail a short-term goal, back up and try again or figure out an alternate root that will get you around the obstacle.

"   When you achieve a short-term goal, celebrate it. Praise yourself liberally as you go along. Psychologists call this reinforcement or rewarding yourself for desired behavior. It is very effective. The reward does not have to be something big. For example, if you are studying for a test, put some nuts or candy on the table. Divide the material you are studying into small units, such as pages, sections of a chapter or basic concepts. As each unit is completed reward yourself with a piece of candy or a nut. It is important to keep the units small and reward yourself frequently. Massive rewards after large amounts of work are less successful. If you try this, you will find studying goes much faster and is more enjoyable. This basic idea can be applied to any task. It is a simple technique that is very effective. This does not mean that you cannot reward yourself for a more major accomplishment. If you complete a course or a semester, treat yourself to an expensive dinner, a short vacation trip, or a gift of some kind. This approach makes getting there half the fun. People who arrange their lives this way enjoy themselves and what they are doing.

Once the long-term and short-term goals have been established, program them into the subconscious using your rules for formulating autosuggestions. After this has been accomplished, do not concentrate on your goals (see Rule VI of Rules of the Mind). If we fix our attention on our goals too firmly, we will find ourselves too future oriented to enjoy the present -- always going somewhere, but never arriving. Looking forward too much to future goals leads us to be unhappy with the present and to make excessive sacrifices to reach our goals. The person that is always concentrating on his future goals is preparing to enjoy the future, and the future never comes. Goals are for direction and planning. After they have been formulated, we need to put them in the back of our mind and begin to concentrate on the present. Remember, a subconscious that is properly programmed can carry out your goals much better than you could ever hope to carry them out consciously.

SELF-INVENTORY

THE OLD ADMONITION, "Know Thy-self," is of the utmost importance. The following list of twenty questions is given to you as a guide only. The aim and purpose you have in learning self-hypnosis may be different than those of someone else. For this reason it is impossible to give specific questions to fit the needs of everyone. None of the following questions may apply to you; they are given to give you an idea of what to look for in yourself.

Self-knowledge is not won without effort. The habits and attitudes you have acquired over many years cannot be changed over night. Some things can be accomplished very quickly and ordinarily the time in self-therapy will not be long. The natural tendency on the part of most students will be to attack their worst problems or conditions first. This is what they are most concerned about. This is a mistake! It is very important to begin with minor matters first. The reason for this is, minor conditions are easier

155

to correct. Success with them encourages you and doubts are eased. As you develop a more positive way of thinking, you will meet less resistance in changing more important conditions.

1. WHAT KIND OF PERSON AM I? You should write a thumbnail sketch of how you see yourself. After you have done that, you should outline that others say you are. For example, if people are always telling you, "My you are moody," write it down. If they say, "You have a nice voice, you should be on radio," write it down. Also, write out how you see yourself physically. Then do the same for how others see you. Do you think what they say is true?

2. WRITE OUT WHAT YOU CONSIDER ARE YOUR GOOD POINTS. "I never lose my temper," or "I am kind to children," or "I always try to help others." If you should feel discouraged while answering any of the following questions, you should refer back to this list. You will find you are really not so bad!

3. DO I GET ALONG WITH MOST PEOPLE? If you are always feuding with others it is a sure indication that you are not getting along with yourself either. You may be projecting the blame on other people, or trying to change other people instead of yourself. Also, you may be over sensitive. When you learn to radiate tolerance, understanding and forgiveness, you will be amazed at how quickly other people's attitudes toward you will change.

4. AM I TOO SHY? Every person is somewhat shy. Even a king. There is a certain normal shyness. It is excessive shyness that is a liability; it blocks you from being yourself as soon as someone else is around. The shy person is afraid he will not be well received and accepted. Shyness is a form of self-protection. If you don't stick your neck out, you can't be hurt. Consequently the shy person becomes uncommunicative and cannot relax around other people. A person that is not overly shy is not too concerned about whether the new person he meets likes him or not. He is realistic. He knows he cannot be liked by everyone. If he experiences situations where he is not liked, he does not necessarily blame himself. He may come to the conclusion that the other person is difficult or expects too much.

Many shy people have handicaps. A stutterer is shy. Somerset Maugham had a stutter, yet it did not stop him from producing some of the greatest literature of his time. If you accept your physical handicaps, others will too. Self-confidence is the antidote to shyness. Structure your suggestions accordingly.

5. AM I SARCASTIC? Sarcasm usually represents over compensation for feeling of insecurity. If you are sarcastic, you are over defensive. You are afraid of being insulted, rejected or disliked by someone, so you beat them to the punch. You act toward a person as you think he might act toward

you. You insult the person you think does not like you, as if to say, "Look, I don't like you either." If you are sarcastic, you are acting out of insecurity. Your job is to build up your own self-image so you will not need to be sarcastic.

6. AM I OVERLY CRITICAL? You are overly critical if you are stingy with your compliments, or are afraid to approve of something, or to say something nice about someone's achievements. Also, you feel you have become a more important person by having something critical to say. If you are overly critical of others, you may have a tendency toward perfectionism. If everything is not just right -- that is, the way you want it -- you are uncomfortable. You are unable to tolerate anyone else doing a thing less perfectly than yourself.

7. DO I POSSESS A DISTORTED SENSE OF VALUES? We are living in a time when emphasis is placed on material things. We are more concerned about being considered successful financially than successful in character. Not that material things are insignificant, but if they have been your major emphasis and you feel unhappy, cheated by life, or as if something is missing, it is a good indication that you need to begin to develop an appreciation for things of the mind. When did you last read a good book, or go to an art gallery?

Sometimes a woman's distorted sense of value may take the form of too great an emphasis on beauty. Becoming more beautiful or staying young can become an obsession. This does not mean that it is not important to look as good as you can, but beauty, when it becomes the end-all of life to the exclusion of improvement of the mind and spirit, leaves the person miserable in spite of beauty. When a man works excessive hours and worries excessively about his business until he has a heart attack, he becomes a victim of his distorted sense of values.

8. DO I SUFFER FROM AN INFERIORITY COMPLEX? To have an inferiority complex is understandable, but to remain inferior is unforgivable and needless. This is one of the easiest conditions to change through self-hypnosis and autosuggestion. Study something that makes you an expert. Gain confidence by doing. Learn to take pride in what you do.

9. AM I ADRIFT WITHOUT GOALS IN LIFE? The saddest people in the world are those who have no goals. They are constantly asking, "What is there to live for?" The woman who is struggling in a poorly paid job to help her son through college will never commit suicide. She has a goal. She is happy and proud. The man or woman who has no responsibilities, who is well paid, and whose only concern is what entertainment he or she can fine for the evening, is much more apt to have a mental break down.

There must be a goal -- a realistic goal that can be obtained. Richard Nixon had a goal; to be President. He failed in it, yet he kept trying. He failed again in a lesser goal, the governorship of California. But the goal still fascinated him, and after years of thinking, planning, and being sustained by his goal, he tried again and won. It had seemed impossible, yet he did it. Most people's goals seem impossible. Who thinks he can write the great American novel? Yet every year books are written by improbable people.

The worst thing that can happen to you is that a little failure makes you so timid you are afraid to dream, afraid to have goals -- big goals. This minute write down the goals that would mean the most to you. Make a list. As many as you like.

What ever your goals are -- start now -- not tomorrow! Study what you need to know, look into problems of going into business for yourself, etc.

10. WHAT WOULD I DO IF I LOST MY JOB? This may seem like a strange question to ask, but you should have an answer. Most people worry now and then -- and some worry excessively -- about what they would do if they were fired or if their job was abolished.

Usually the worst does not happen. But, the response to fear is to have an answer, an alternative. White down what you would do if you did receive that pink slip. Make out a list of the places you would go to find another job and perhaps a better job. Jot down things you could do to earn some money while you were waiting for a job to come through. If you do not have any side skills, isn't it time that you developed some?

11. AM I OVER SENSITIVE? If you are, you probably feel that no one should disagree with you. That is, no one has the right to be careless of your feelings. In other words, you are vain. You have to be practical. Even a rose comes to you with thorns on it. So does life, full of thorns. You cannot say the rose is no good, or life is no good because of the thorns. To be practical, you must tell yourself that people are going to be careless of your feelings, sometimes intentionally and sometimes unintentionally. What can you do about it? You can desensitize yourself and promise yourself that no one can demoralize you or make you lose confidence in yourself.

12. AM I TOO CONCEITED? People who are conceited are covering up for an inferiority complex. A person who has achieved great things has no need to feel conceited. Almost without exception, great people are humble and modest. People who are conceited lose friends rapidly. They make themselves obnoxious. They are always pointing out subtly or bluntly how much better they are than other people. They tend to display all kinds of prejudices that are their way of pointing out how superior they are.

13. AM I IMMATURE? The immature person has the traits of a child who has not learned to control his or her desires, emotions and thinking. They are selfish, lack emotional control and wise

158

judgment. They want everything their way. They sulk and pout. In other words, they do what you would expect a very young child to do.

Being mature, on the other hand, is synonymous with being wise, acting with wisdom, exercising self-control, and thinking things through without too much emotion. It means showing tolerance and understanding -- knowing how the other person feels and explaining why you are taking the position you are.

14. AM I A CHRONIC COMPLAINER? The chronic complainer is sabotaging both his physical and his mental health. He becomes a hypochondriac. He believes everyone is against him or perhaps the world has singled him out for all its bad luck. The chronic complainer will find justification for each complaint. He will finally conclude, no one understands him and no one is on his side. Chronic complainers are unhappy people. They will overlook a multitude of good things to find one flaw. This is not to say, there are not situations in life when it is necessary to offer constructive suggestions. But you must distinguish between normal complaining that is reasonable, and neurotic, excessive and unreasonable complaining whereby a person complains for the sake of complaining.

15. DO I ACT LIKE A SPENDTHRIFT OR A STINGY PERSON? If you are either, you are suffering from insecurity. Persons who are frustrated, who have not found love, may be reckless with money. They buy what ever they see and like, whether they can afford it or not. People who are always in debt are disorganized in their thinking. They handle money like they handle their emotions.

Borrowers of money want something from other people. They want others to support them, as it they were entitled to it. They do not want to assume the responsibility of earning their own way through life. They like to involve other people in their problems. This is a substitute for their search for love.

Persons who are over generous to a fault may be inspired by a desire to buy the love of other people. They want to be well thought of. They want everyone indebted to them in an effort to keep their friendship.

The person who cannot give anything to anyone, who is called a skinflint by those who know him, cannot give anything else of value either, especially love. He cannot get over the hurt he has suffered, generally in childhood, of not receiving enough love himself. Now he is bitter and will not give love, or material things.

16. DO I HARBOR STRONG PREJUDICES? What has been said about people that are conceited applies to persons who are prejudiced. It is evidence of their own insecurity. Individuals that have strong prejudices achieve a false sense of superiority by believing they are better than some other

159

person or group of people. Prejudice is also a cover up for fear and jealousy. We become prejudiced against people we fear, people whom we believe may threaten our own sense of security.

Prejudice leads to hatred, which in turn causes a person to become emotionally disturbed. You become the victim of hate, much more than the thing hated. Prejudice is the product of false thinking. You can have likes and dislikes without making blanket prejudices of them that are unreasonable and only hurt yourself.

17. DO I WORRY TOO MUCH? Worrying to excess is a habit that is learned. Habits are not inherited. You were not born to worry. Like all bad habits, the worry habit can be de-conditioned. Develop a feeling of emotional self-confidence, a belief in yourself and any worry will disappear.

The rest of the questions are given without comment. Think about them and decide it they are problems that are keeping you from achieving happiness. You may have other areas you would like to work on. If so, write them down.

18. DO I DRINK TOO MUCH?

19. AM I LIVING IN THE PAST?

20. DO I HAVE MORBID FEARS?

YOU CAN LEARN TO RELAX

This is a tense world, as many of us well know. We talk about "tension" and we read about it. It is discussed on the radio and on T.V. It is written about in books, newspapers and magazine articles. There is a growing realization of something excessive in our way of living that can lead to disorder and malady.

As the pace of modern living continues to increase, almost every individual is obliged to meet demands on their nervous energy that would not have been made many years ago. As a remedy we are told to "take it easy, relax." However, most people are so busy living their daily lives that they rarely, if ever, allow themselves the opportunity of experiencing total relaxation. Many people claim that they "relax" by driving, playing golf, collecting stamps or by some other hobby. But, what they mean by relaxation is vague even in their own minds.

The real problem is that most people simply do not know how to relax. This is very unfortunate because the ability to relax in any situation is a tremendously valuable skill that anyone can learn in a very short period of time. Once the skill is developed, it is possible to remain calm and at ease in situations that normally produce anxiety or tension. For example, many individuals become tense or anxious when they meet new people, when they are in a strange or new situation and when they feel that they are being judged by others. Individuals who drink excessively, or who may be trying to quit smoking, become very tense and anxious when they have not had their usual drink, snack, or cigarette. Some individuals experience great anxiety in certain specific situations such as riding in airplanes, being in closed areas or in high places, etc. If these individuals could just learn to relax in the stressful situations, they could control or completely eliminate their anxiety.

Modern research has shown that "inner tension" depends for its survival on existing in a vicious circle. The circle may begin with fear, anxiety, or over stimulation and can build to include such elements as frustration, sleeplessness, fatigue, talkativeness, anger, etc. But one part of the circle that is always present is muscle tension. Relax those tense muscles and you break the circle. It is absolutely impossible to feel angry, fearful, anxious, insecure or "unsafe" as long as your muscles remain perfectly relaxed. Tension in muscles is a "preparation for action" -- or a "getting ready to respond." Relaxation of muscles brings about "mental relaxation," or a peaceful "relaxed attitude."

Tension is a rather vague word when it is used to describe inner feelings and emotions. But, muscle tension is a definite physical thing. Make a tight fist and note the tension. That is muscle tension. Now let your hand slowly turn limp. That is relaxation. The more slowly you loosen the fist to final limpness, the more surely you may identify the feeling of limpness, the more surely you may identify the feeling of relaxation happening -- and your control of it. Squint your eyes tightly shut and compress your lips. Slowly let them go limp. Get the feel of it.

If you train yourself over a period of time to repeat these simple exercises, first with the large, easily controlled muscles, then with the smaller ones whose tensions are subtler, you will find it possible to relax at will, all the way down to a repose quieter than normal sleep.

Thousands who have learned to calm "uncontrollable" tensions by relaxing controllable muscles find it works every time. But it takes practice, a willingness to keep at it. The process is progressive, not instantaneous. For every minute that you keep the larger muscles relaxed, more of the smaller ones will let go -- even if you haven't yet the skill to relax the small ones voluntarily. If you are either exceedingly or subtly tense, and as yet unskilled in the fine points, you are not likely to be wholly calm after five or ten minutes of partial relaxation. The process is like turning off all the lights -- the house won't be dark until the last switch is thrown.

Here are some things that you can begin to do immediately to help you to achieve a "relaxed feeling" and "relaxed attitude" while going about your daily activities:

" Keep your hands and arms limp when not in use.

" Keep your face -- especially your lips and brows -- placid when not talking and no more activity than necessary when talking.

" Let your shoulders hang on their bones unless they have a load to bear.

" Let go any needless rigidity in your legs and feet when they aren't carrying you.

If you do these four things, you will find a pleasant change toward serenity creeping up on you.

Try this: catch yourself, if you can, in moments of pressure, excitement, hurry, argument. Notice the muscle tension that always goes with them. Now relax every one of those muscles that you can without falling down or looking ridiculous. Maintain all the muscular relaxation you can while still playing your role in the situation. Try it 40 times, not just once. Then you be the judge of what seems to happen to your part of the tenseness of the situation.

No matter what you do in daily life, you will do it better, with less fatigue and better judgment, if you "hang loose." As you habitually relax needless tensions in your voluntary muscles, this state of relaxation will spread even to muscles that are not directly controllable, such as those involved in stomach tensions (Which is something to think about if you work under pressure that has your stomach "tightening up in knots").

As a part of this course you will be taught a method for inducing a very profound state of physical relaxation using words and visual imagery. As you continue your daily practice, begin to form a habit of mentally remembering the pleasant relaxed feeling that you induced. Stop occasionally during the day, it need only take a moment, and remember in detail the sensations of relaxation. Remember how your arms felt, your legs, back, neck and face. Sometimes forming a mental picture of yourself lying in bed, or sitting relaxed and limp in an easy chair helps to recall the relaxed sensations. Mentally repeating to yourself several times, "I feel more and more relaxed," also helps. Practice this remembering faithfully several times each day. You will be surprised at how much it reduces fatigue and how much better you are able to handle situations. In time, your relaxed attitude will become a habit, and you will no longer need to consciously practice it.

GLOSSARY OF TERMS

Abstraction: Process of developing concepts; that is, grouping objects in terms of some distinguishing common property.

Acetylcholine: A neurotransmitter. In the brain it helps regulate memory. In the peripheral nervous system, controls the actions of skeletal and smooth muscle.

Action Potential: An electrical potential that occurs when a neuron is activated and temporarily reverses the electrical state of its interior membrane from negative to positive. This electrical charge

162

travels along the axon to the neuron's terminal where it triggers or inhibits the release of a neurotransmitter.

Afferent Neuron: Neuron that carries messages toward the central nervous system from a receptor cell. Also known as a sensory neuron.

All-Or-Nothing Law: Principle that if a nerve fiber responds at all, it responds with full strength.

Alpha Rhythms: The electrical rhythm typical of the brain during normal wakefulness. About 8 to 12 oscillations per second.

Amino Acid Transmitters: The most prevalent neurotransmitters in the brain, these include glutamate and aspartate, which have excitatory actions, and glycine and gamma-amino butyric acid (GABA) which have inhibitory actions.

Amnesia: Loss of memory; it can be total or partial.

Analgesia: Absence of the sense of pain.

Aphasia: Disturbance in language comprehension or production.

Auditory Nerve: A bundle of nerve fibers extending from the cochlea of the ear to the brain, which contains two branches: the cochlear nerve that transmits sound information and the vestibular nerve that relays information related to balance.

Auto Rotatory Movements: The impossibility to stop a rotatory movement (generally of the forearms) once it has been started by the hypnotist.

Automatic Writing: The unconscious action of writing, performed in a state of trance.

Autonomic Nervous System (ANS:) That part of the nervous system that regulates bodily activities not ordinarily subject to voluntary control. Its activities are divided between the sympathetic and parasympathetic divisions.

Autosuggestion: The action of giving oneself suggestions.

Axon: The fiber like extension of a neuron by which the cell sends information to target cells.

Behavior: The activity of organisms.

Beta Rhythms: Rhythms in the EEG of a frequency of about 25 per second.

Bodily Image: The person's perception of himself.

Brain: The central nervous system above the spinal cord.

Brainstem: The major route by which the forebrain sends information to and receives information from the spinal cord and peripheral nerves. It controls, among other things, respiration and regulation of heart rhythms.

Broca's Area: The brain region located in the frontal lobe of the left hemisphere that is important for the production of speech.

Catalepsy: A state in which the subject has no external sensitivity and cannot perform voluntary movements. It is usually manifested by a rigidity of the body or certain parts of the body. In this condition the body and the limbs will keep any position in which they are placed.

Central Nervous System (CNS): That portion of the nervous system that lies within the skull and spinal column; the brain and spinal cord.

Cerebral Cortex: The part of the brain associated with conscious experience and higher mental processes. A grayish rind of tissue covering the cerebrum.

Cerebral hemispheres: They are symmetrical halves of the brain. There are two occipital lobes, two parietal lobes and two frontal lobes. These two hemispheres are in continual communication with one other. Each functions as an independent parallel processor with complementary functions.

Cerebrum: The main part of man's brain, divided into right and left hemispheres; also known as the new brain.

Cognition: The process or processes by which an organism gains knowledge of or becomes aware of events or objects in its environment and uses that knowledge for comprehension and problem-solving.

Conditioned Reflex (Response) (CR): A learned response to a stimulus not originally capable of arousing the response.

Conditioned Stimulus (CS): A stimulus, ordinarily ineffective, which by association with an unconditioned stimulus becomes effective in eliciting behavior.

Conditioning: Basic form of learning in which conditioned responses are established.

Cone: A primary receptor cell for vision located in the retina. It is sensitive to color and used primarily for daytime vision.

Consciousness: A term used to describe an individual organism while it is perceiving, remembering, thinking, imagining, etc.

Cornea: A thin, curved transparent membrane on the surface of the front of the eye. It begins the focusing process for vision.

Cortex: This is where most high-level functions associated with the mind are implemented. Some of its regions are highly specialized. For example, the motor cortex helps coordinate all voluntary muscle movements. The occipital lobes located near the rear of the brain interprets visual stimuli.

Covert: An adjective applied to internal activities of organisms that ordinarily can be observed only with the aid of special instruments.

Delta Rhythms: Rather slow rhythms in the EEG, characteristic of light sleep.

Dendrite: A tree-like extension of the neuron cell body. Along with the cell body, it receives information from other neurons.

Dissociation*: Normally the recalling of memories is a result of the association of ideas. If there is a failure in the ability to recall events, which normally should be remembered, it is termed "dissociation" -- an interruption of the memory.

Dissociation of Awareness*: A selective constriction of awareness, which excludes all sources of stimulation, except for the suggestions of the hypnotist.

Effectors: The organs (muscles or glands) that perform the actual response functions of adjustment.

Efferent Neurons: Neuron that carries messages from the CNS to an organ of response. Also known as motor neuron.

Emotion: Internal or visceral activity.

Emotional Behavior: Behavior that is activated by the ANS.

165

Endorphins: Neurotransmitters produced in the brain that generate cellular and behavioral effects like those of morphine.

Epinephrine: A hormone, released by the adrenal medulla and the brain that acts with norepinephrine to activate the sympathetic division of the autonomic nervous system. Sometimes called adrenaline.

Evoked Potentials: A measure of the brain's electrical activity in response to sensory stimuli. This is obtained by placing electrodes on the surface of the scalp (or more rarely, inside the head), repeatedly administering a stimulus, and then using a computer to average the results.

Excitation: A change in the electrical state of a neuron that is associated with an enhanced probability of action potentials.

Forebrain: The largest division of the brain, which includes the cerebral cortex and basal ganglia. It is credited with the highest intellectual functions.

Frontal lobes: Located behind the forehead. They are most closely linked with making decisions and judgments.

Galvanic Skin Response (GSR): Increase in voltage and/or change in electrical resistance of the skin occurring during emotion as a result of action of the ANS on the sweat glands.

Gamma-Amino Butyric Acid (GABA): An amino acid transmitter in the brain whose primary function is to inhibit the firing of neurons.

Gastrointestinal Tract: The digestive tract, from mouth to anus.

Glia: Specialized cells that nourish and support neurons.

Glutamate: An amino acid neurotransmitter that acts to excite neurons. Glutamate probably stimulates N-methyl-D-aspartate (NMDA) receptors that have been implicated in activities ranging from learning and memory to development and specification of nerve contacts in a developing animal. Stimulation of NMDA receptors may promote beneficial changes; while over stimulation may be the cause of nerve cell damage or death in neurological trauma and stroke.

Hallucination: Sensory impression of external objects in the absence of external stimulus.

Hetroaction: A progressively increasing tendency of an individual to respond to other suggestions after being made to respond to a number of previous suggestions. A generalization of suggestibility.

Hippocampus: This area plays a crucial role in processing information involving long-term memory. Damage to the hippocampus will produce global retrograde amnesia, or the inability to store information.

Homoaction: The tendency of an ideomotor response to increase in strength if it is elicited a number of times within a certain interval of time. Homoaction accumulates with multiple repetitions of a suggestion.

Homeostasis: The tendency of organisms to maintain internal equilibrium.

Hormones: Chemical messengers secreted by endocrine glands to regulate the activity of target cells. They play a role in sexual development, calcium and bone metabolism, growth and many other activities.

Hyperhydrosis: Excessive perspiration, usually from the hands, feet and armpits.

Hypnosis: A normal state of the nervous system that is characterized by increased suggestibility.

Hypnotic Regression: Process, by which a subject vividly relives, under hypnosis, experiences which he has forgotten or repressed.

Hypnoidal: The state in which the first effects of hypnosis are felt.

Ideomotor Response: A muscular or motor response to an idea held in the mind.

Imagery: Includes responses in all sensory classifications. Imagery is not all visual. It is possible to imagine, in varying degrees, other kinds of sensory impressions (sounds, odor, taste, touch, etc.).

Immediate Memory: A phase of memory that is extremely short-lived, with information stored only for a few seconds. It also is known as short-term and working memory.

Inhibition: In reference to neurons, it is a synaptic message that prevents the recipient cell from firing.

Kinesthesis: Muscle, tendon and joint sensitivities.

Left Cerebral Hemisphere: This part of the brain is most closely associated with consciousness. The left hemisphere usually manages the right side of the body, controls language and general cognitive functions. It plays a predominate role in deciding what responses are made to incoming stimuli.

Limbic system: Contains a number of interconnected brain structures which are linked to hormones, drives, temperature control, emotion, and, to memory formation. Neurons affecting heart rate and respiration are concentrated in the hypothalamus and direct most of the physiological changes that accompany strong emotion.

Long-Term Memory: The final phase of memory in which information storage may last from hours to a lifetime.

Neuron: Individual nerve cell.

Neuro-Semantics: The science of the effect that words have on the human nervous system.

Mania: A mental disorder characterized by excessive excitement. A form of psychosis with exalted feelings, delusions of grandeur, elevated mood, psychomotor over activity and overproduction of ideas.

Memory Consolidation: The physical and psychological changes that take place as the brain organizes and restructures information in order to make it a permanent part of memory.

Monoideism: The domination of the nervous system by one single idea.

Motor Neuron: A neuron that carries information from the central nervous system to the muscle.

Myelin: Compact fatty material that surrounds and insulates axons of some neurons.

Neuron: Nerve cell. It is specialized for the transmission of information and characterized by long fibrous projections called axons, and shorter, branch-like projections called dendrites.

Neurotransmitter: A chemical released by neurons at a synapse for the purpose of relaying information by way of receptors.

Overt: An adjective applied to behavior that can be observed without the aid of special instruments.

Parasympathetic Nervous System (PNS): That portion of the ANS that controls most of the ordinary vital functions of life, such as digestion. Its action is antithetic to that of the sympathetic division in most cases.

Parietal Lobe: One of the four subdivisions of the cerebral cortex. It plays a role in sensory processes, attention and language.

Perception: The interpretation of sensation. Process of becoming aware of objects, events, and qualities that stimulate the sense organs and of determining the relationship between them.

Peripheral Nervous System: A division of the nervous system consisting of all nerves not part of the brain or spinal cord.

Placebo: A sham drug having no physiological effect, used in research to avoid the factor of suggestion.

Post-Hypnotic Suggestion: Suggestion that becomes or remains active after the hypnotic session is over.

Psychosomatic disorder: A physical disorder believed to be of psychogenic origin.

Receptor: A cell differentiated from others in terms of its increased irritability to certain stimuli.

Receptor Molecule: A specific molecule on the surface or inside of a cell with a characteristic chemical and physical structure. Many neurotransmitters and hormones exert their effects by binding to receptors on cells.

Reciprocal Innervation: The balance of impulses leading to the relaxation of one of a pair of antagonistic muscles as the other contracts.

Reflex: A relative simple, innate response to a particular stimulus.

Reflex Arc: Simplest neural link from receptor to effector involving the CNS. Consists of a receptor, afferent neuron, sometimes a connection neuron or neurons, efferent neuron and effector.

Regression: The state induced by hypnosis in which a subject relives a previous period of his life.

Right cerebral hemisphere: Controls the left half of the body. In most people it manages nonverbal processes, such as attention, pattern recognition, line orientation and the detection of complex auditory tones.

Rod: A sensory neuron located in the periphery of the retina. It is sensitive to light of low intensity and specialized for nighttime vision.

Semantics: Technique for sharpening the accuracy of thinking; emphasizes the need for operational definitions of words and the importance of avoiding the tendency to regard words as things rather than as mere names for concepts.

Semantic Conditioning: Refers to the formation of conditioned responses to the meanings of verbal stimuli rather than their physical attributes (i.e. the sound of a word).

Sensation: The un-interpreted experience accompanying afferent activity that reaches the cortical level.

Sensitization: A change in behavior or biological response by an organism that is produced by delivering a strong, generally noxious, stimulus.

Short-Term Memory: A phase of memory in which a limited amount of information may be held for several seconds to minutes.

Stimulus: A change brought about in a receptor by a signal from the environment.

Symbol: An image, object or activity that represents and can be substituted for something else. For example, words and numbers.

Sympathetic Nervous System (SNS): Division of the ANS that is active in emergency conditions of extreme cold, violent effort or exercise and states of fear or rage.

Synapse: A gap between two neurons that functions as the site of information transfer from one neuron to another.

Suggestion: An idea conveyed to the mind by an action or through the spoken word.

Temporal Lobe: One of the four major subdivisions of each hemisphere of the cerebral cortex. It functions in auditory perception, speech and complex visual perceptions.

Thalamus: A structure consisting of two egg-shaped masses of nerve tissue, each about the size of a walnut, deep within the brain. It is the key relay station for sensory information flowing into the brain, filtering out only information of particular importance from the mass of signals entering the brain.

Trance: A particular state of the nervous system obtained in hypnosis. By extension, every hypnotic state: light trance, medium trance, deep trance, etc.

Unconditioned Reflex (Response) (UR): A response that occurs to appropriate stimulation without prior conditioning.

Unconditioned Stimulus (US): A stimulus that affects behavior without prior learning.

Wernicke's Area: A region of the brain responsible for the comprehension of language and the production of meaningful speech.

*The concept of dissociation is widely used, but poorly defined. By "dissociation of awareness" we mean a separation or segregation off from awareness of a group of mental processes. In the induction of hypnosis there is apparently a stage during which consciousness is highly constricted, that is dissociated from that which would normally constitute its content.

The 12 Devices That Almost Instantly Hypnotize

Published by Velocity Group Publishing

PO Box 9516 Hamilton, NJ 08650   www.advancedmindpower.com   www.mindforcesecrets.com
© Copyright 2008   All Rights Reserved

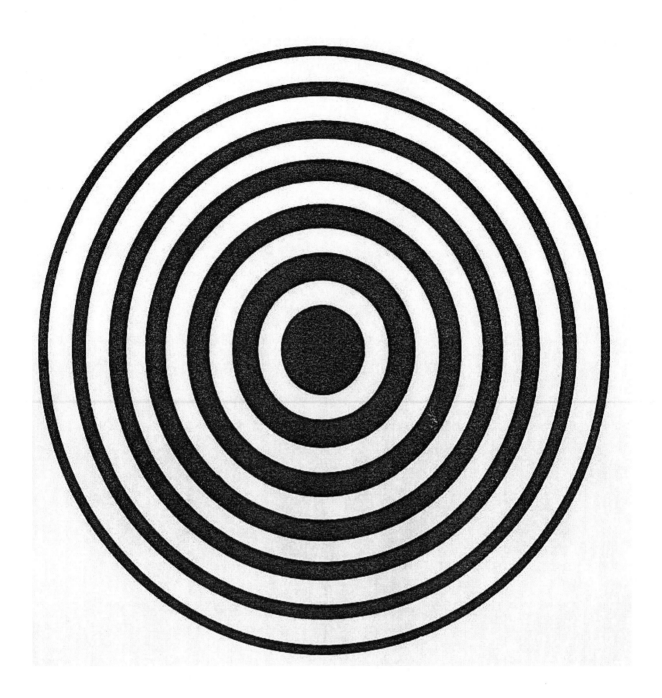

174

Preface

In this booklet you will find preliminary methods that will build your hypnotic power and develop your personal magnetism.

These "secret" devices- some of them revealed to the public for the first time- And only valid with training. Do not try to judge them in advance, put them into practice. It works by practicing- and practicing alone. Then you will obtain the results you desire.

1- BE PREPARED

One of the devices for hypnotic power resides in the hypnotist's physical and mental preparation.

From a physical viewpoint, food that is hard to digest, alcohol and tobacco should be kept in moderation. In general, anything that tends to interfere with or weaken concentration is detrimental to your hypnotic power.

Staying in good physical condition and sleeping well facilitate the practice of hypnotism. For mental preparation, start by reading and rereading the following phrases every day:

I want to

I can

I am sure of myself

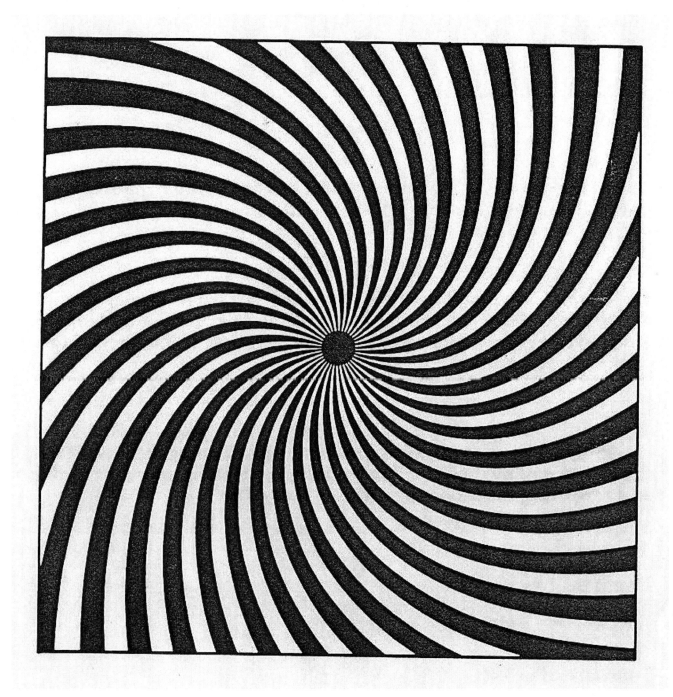

2- DEVELOP THE INTENSITY OF YOUR GAZE

Place the design on the opposite page about 11 inches away from your eyes, slightly above eye level. Start by fixating on the black circle in the middle. If you feel your attention wandering at first, close your eyes for a few seconds and begin again, always fixating on the center of the circle.

Try to keep your eyes open as long a possible without blinking. After a few minutes you will see the circle divide into two points that gradually move two inches or so apart while you begin to feel more and more relaxed and fixated on the circle. This marks the start of auto-hypnotism.

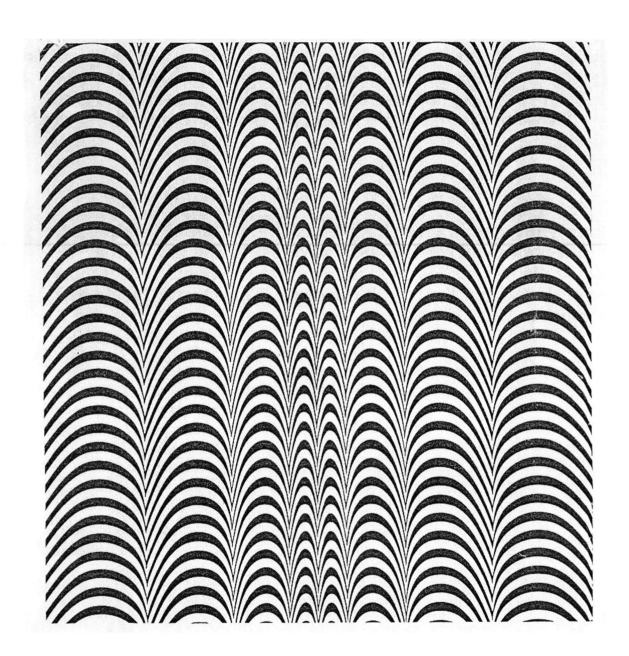

180

3- PRACTICE AUTOSUGGESTION

Once you have reached this state of calmness and relaxation, concentrate on the following phrases, one after the other, repeating them to yourself:

I feel my will grow stronger and stronger

My hypnotic power develops day by day

No one can resist the power of my gaze

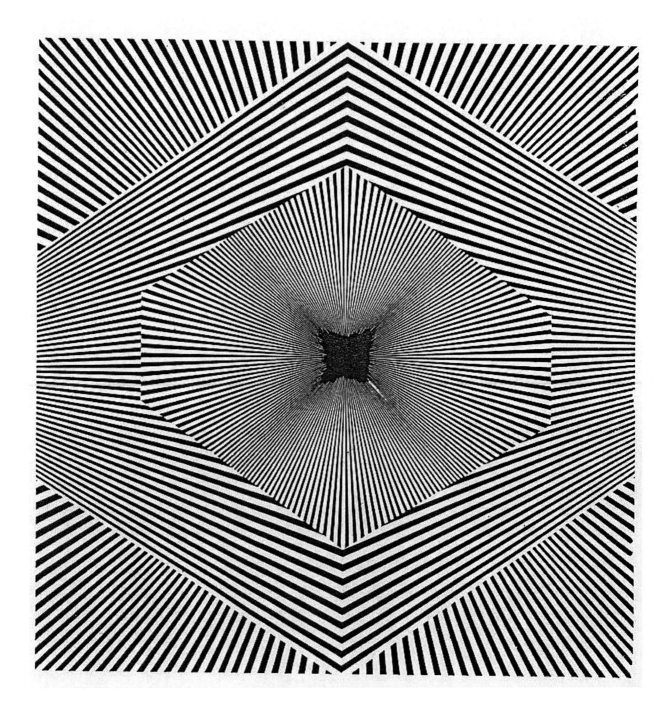

4- BUILD UP YOUR ENERGY

Breathe calmly, using your diaphragm and abdominal muscles, and with each inhalation mentally envision yourself taking in cosmic energy. Every time you exhale, project the accumulated energy through your eyes. Imagine that energy surrounding your subject, enveloping him or her in the power of your magnetism.

You can think of your fluid as a violet-colored ray.

Note that the longer you do this exercise the more powerful your fluid and energy becomes.

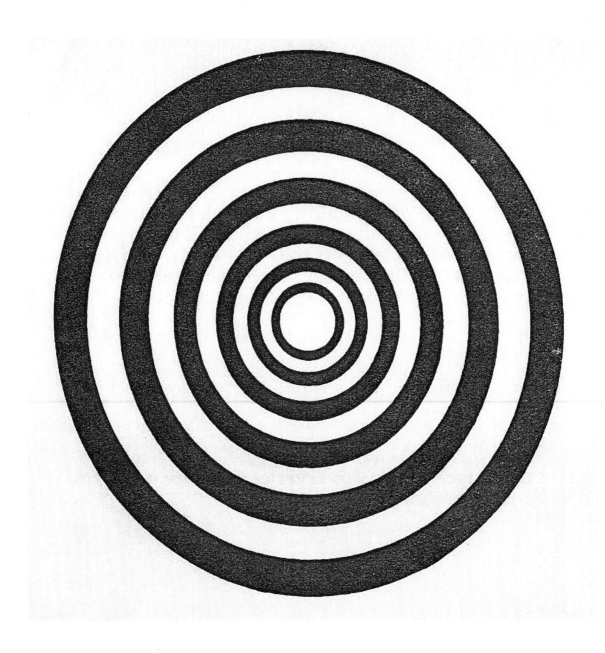

5- HOW TO HYPNOTIZE EASILY

Take one of the hypnotic designs in this booklet and hold it 10 or 12 inches away from the subject, high enough from his forehead that he must make an effort with his eyes and eyelids.

Ask the subject to fixate his eyes on concentrate his mind exclusively on the design. The subjects pupils will contract, at first, then dilate. Once they dilate, move your hand close to his eyes. His eyelids will close involuntarily in a vibratory movement.

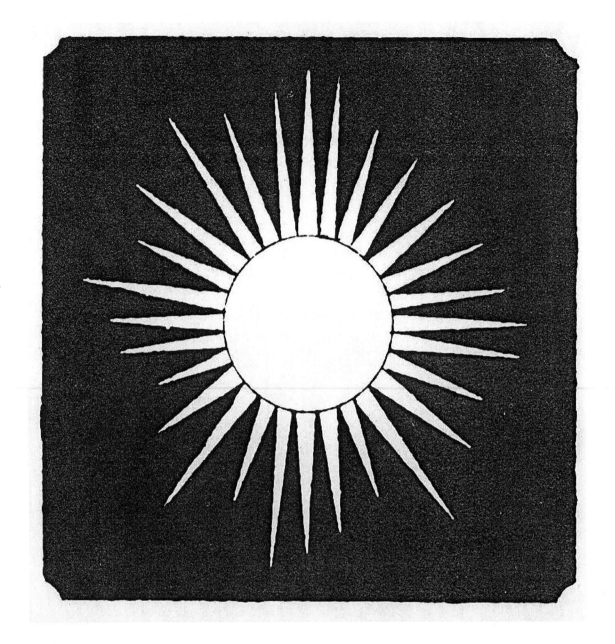

6- REINFORCE THE EFFECT THROUGH SUGGESTION

If the subject does not shut his eyes, start again, asking him to do so as you approach your hand.

You can reinforce the effect by saying the following:

"Remain tranquil and serene. Your eyes are fixated on the center of this design. Nothing else exists. Your entire universe is concentrated on this point, nothing else. Keep your eyes focused on the center of this design...."

Then you continue with the suggestions that you feel are necessary for him or her

187

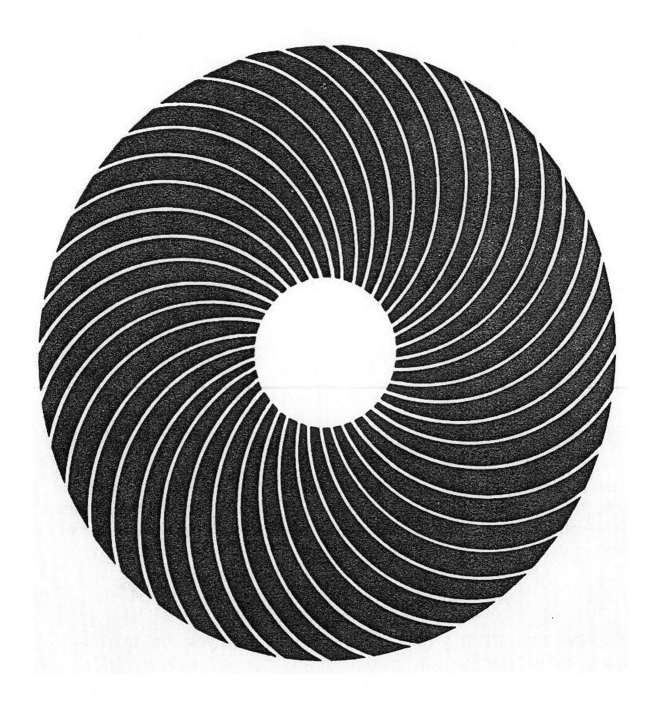

7- ROTATE THE DESIGN

Slow, circular movement of the design will enhance the effect. You also can use any rotary mechanism. In that case, the spiral will give the best results.

8- UTILIZE THE "MIRROR EFFECT"

Tape one of the designs in this booklet on a large mirror.

Ask the subject to fixate on the design until he is no longer aware of his own image.

Or you can ask him instead to alternate-to concentrate his attention on the design for 30 seconds, then on the environment, then back to the design.

This is also excellent training for auto-hypnotism.

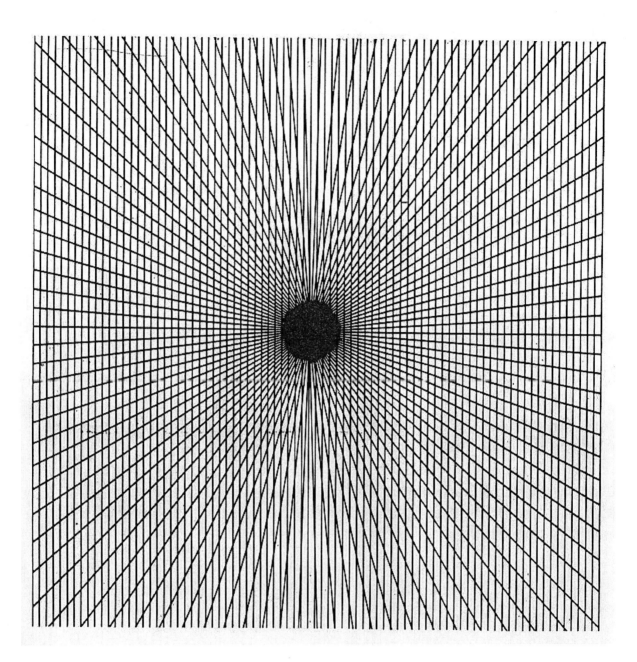

9- DEVICES FOR DEVELOPING A POTENT GAZE

We have already seen one of them: Its intensity. The second is the exact point where the subject should be fixated. That point is located PRECISELY BETWEEN THE EYES, in other words, at the root of the nose. This point is sometimes referred to as "The Third Eye".

While projecting the power of your gaze, you can picture what you want mentally: create an image of your subject already asleep and think of the phrases that induce hypnosis as described in this method.

Often, by following this procedure, you can put someone to sleep without saying a word, just by simple fixation and telepathic suggestion.

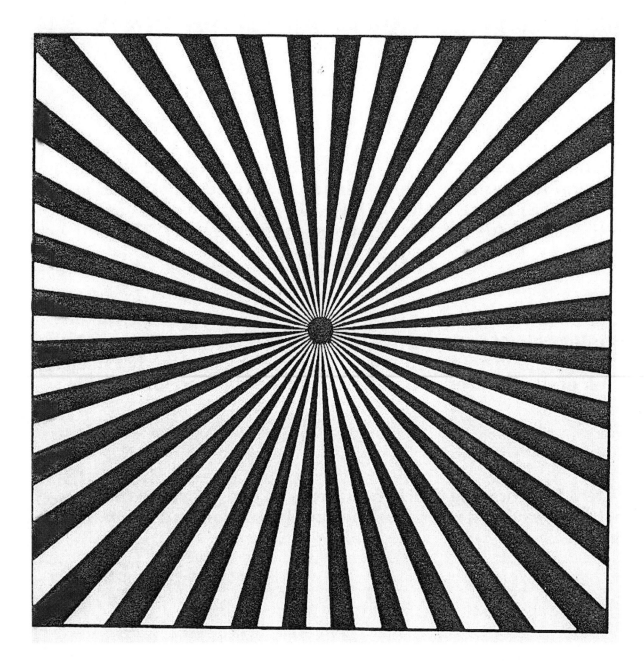

10-USE YOUR HANDS AS TRANSMITTERS

Much like your gaze, your hands are powerful sources of magnetic influence.

Point your fingers toward the subject, toward his temples especially, and you will hypnotize him easier.

You can actually " energy charge" the hypnotic drawing shown here as a fixation point.

To do this, Inhale, take in energy, and send your force toward the design as you exhale.

FINAL ADVICE

The ideal way to almost instantly hypnotize is to accumulate the effect of gaze, magnetism, hypnotic designs, voice and gestures. This cumulative effect will guarantee you maximum success in all situations.

Some Closing Thoughts

This bonus volume of Mind Force Hypnosis: Closed Door Hypnosis Files, should have given you all the pieces to your Hypnotic puzzle. It is always my intention to provide excellent material for you to enhance your skills and the books contained in this volume do exactly that.

Respectfully,

A. Thomas Perhacs, Publisher

www.mindforcesecrets.com

www.advancedmindpower.com

www.chipower.com

My Other Products

Manipulation

Mind Force Hypnosis

Chi Power Plus

Mind Portal

Magneto

Power of the Mind

Closed Door Hypnosis Files

Advanced Chi DVD

Dim Mak Striking

The Goal Setting Formula

Chi Power Inner Circle Membership

CPSIA information can be obtained at www.ICGtesting.com
Printed in the USA
BVOW05s2035111113

336032BV00002B/58/P